HAKKA

KWONGSAI SOUTHERN

MANTIS

PICTORIAL BOOK
OF BOXING
POSTURES & MAXIMS

PICTORIAL OF BOXING

Bamboo Temple Chinese Benevolent Association
Featured in this Book
Wong Bak Lim (L), RDH (R)
circa 1992, New York Chinatown

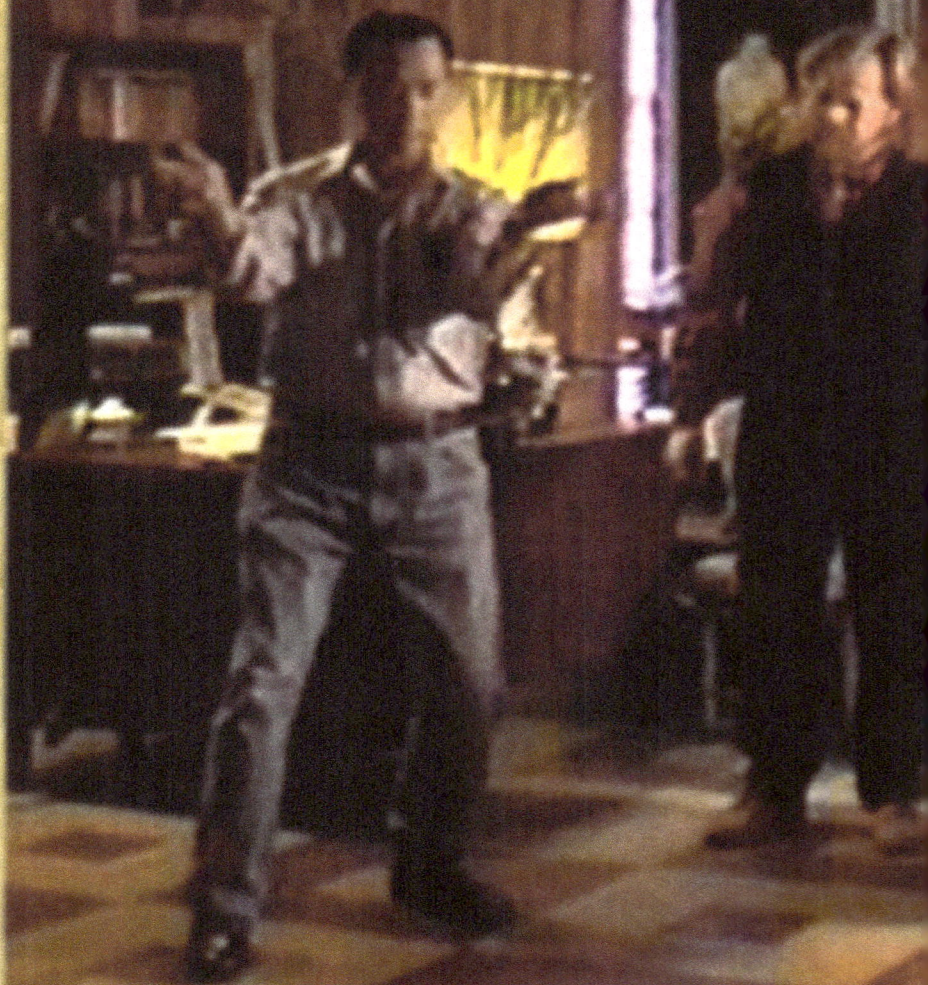

Southern Mantis Press

POSTURES & MAXIMS

Bamboo Temple Association
Founded Circa 1963,
New York City

Sifu Wong Bak Lim,
Master Lam Sang's
first inner gate
disciple, founded
the Bamboo Temple
Chinese Benevolent
Association. The
announcement
and photo below
was featured in
 the local
Chinatown
newspapers
and Chinese
 media. Today,
we continue to
carry forward
this legacy
some sixty years
later.

L) Jesse Eng Sibok
R) Harry Sun Sibok

China Hakka Mantis Series

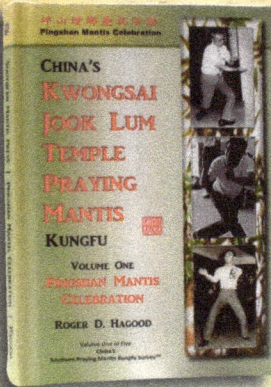

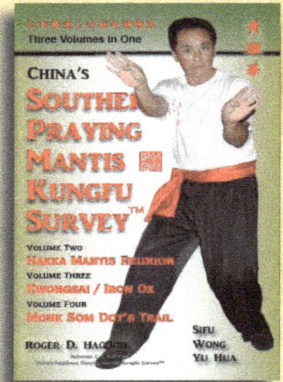

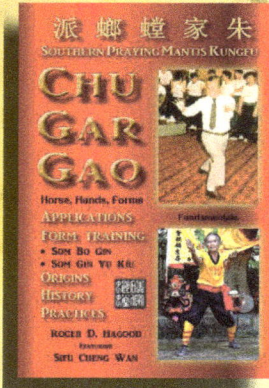

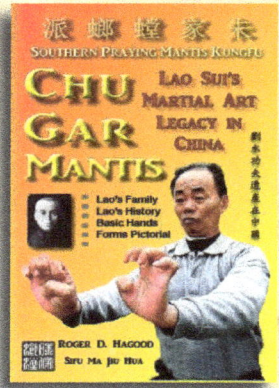

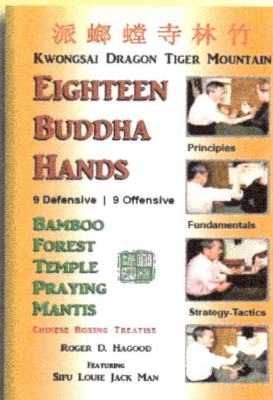

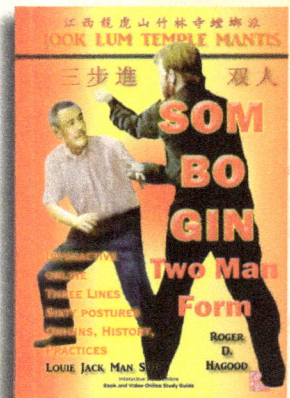

HAKKA

KWONGSAI SOUTHERN

MANTIS

PICTORIAL BOOK OF
BOXING POSTURES AND MAXIMS

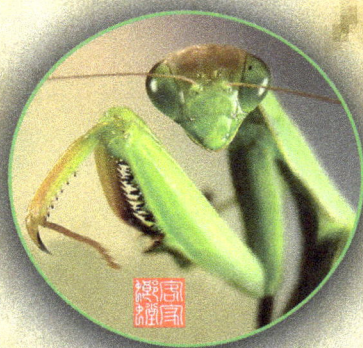

By

Roger D. Hagood

Demonstrated by the
Bamboo Temple Chinese Benevolent Association

Editors
Charles Alan Clemens, Sean W. Robinson, Huang Yan

Southern Mantis Press | Pingshan Town, China

Southern Mantis Press
5424 NW Cascade Court
Camas, WA 98607
books@southernmantispress.com

Ordering Information:
Special discounts are available for martial art schools, bookstores, specialty shops, museums and events.   Contact the publisher at the email address above.

ISBN: 978-0-9857240-9-2

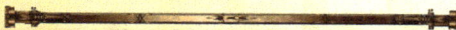

Dedication

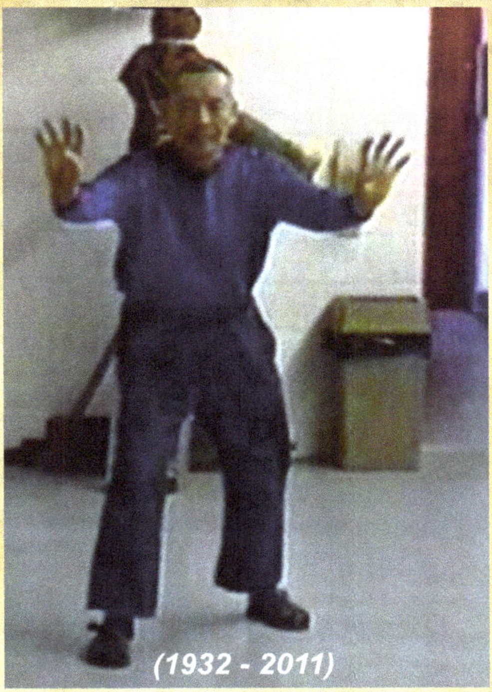

(1932 - 2011)

Louie Jack Man

Louie Sifu cared about Southern Praying Mantis Kungfu. My great regret is that I did not complete the *"Eighteen Buddha Hands"* book before he passed. We made pictures for that book in the late 1990s. He had the manuscript for the book back then too, and his mood always seemed to improve when we discussed the book. Though he passed in 2011, we can still remember and benefit from his teaching now.

mantisflix.com

Acknowledgement

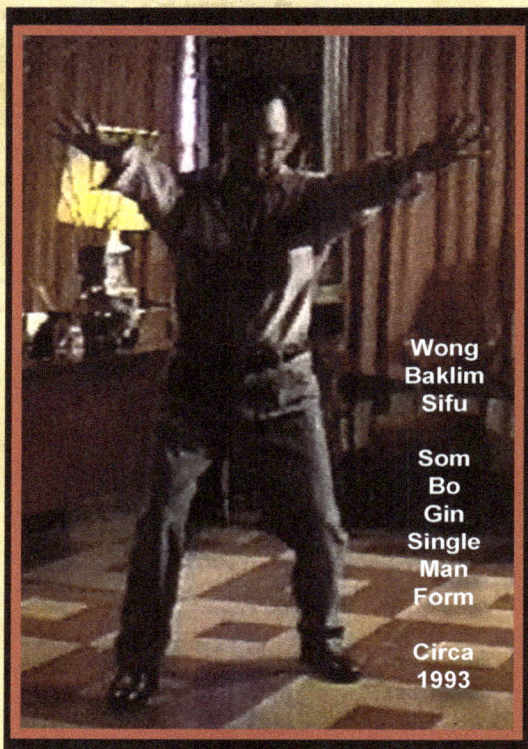

Wong
Baklim
Sifu

Som
Bo
Gin
Single
Man
Form

Circa
1993

Sibok Wong Baklim

This book features members of the Bamboo Temple Chinese Benevolent Association and so it is appropriately co-dedicated to Wong Baklim. Wong Sifu is the "dai-sihing," the first disciple that Grand Sifu Lam Sang accepted, in the 1950s USA. Wong Sifu founded the Bamboo Temple Chinese Benevolent Association circa 1963, in New York City, to preserve and promote Lam Sang's teaching. After more than 20 years of brother-friendship with Wong Sifu and Uncles Eng and Sun Sibok, the tradition carries onward.

Our Ancestral Shrine

Southern Praying Mantis Kungfu Creed

Hoc Yurn; Hoc Yi; Hoc Kungfu

學仁　學義　學功夫

Jurn Jow; Jurn Si; Jurn Gow Do

尊親　尊師　尊教訓　尊道義

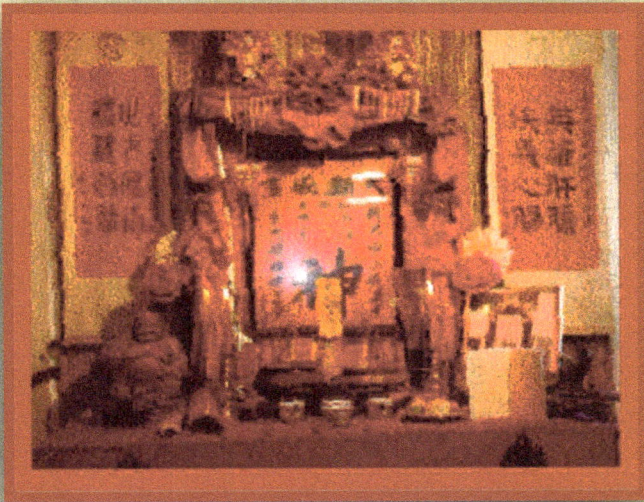

Respect the Ancestors for their
transmission of the art.

Respect the Sifu for his teaching.

Respect the Older Brothers for their
dedication and loyalty.

Respect the Younger Brothers for
determination in training.

Contents

Front Matter

Pictorial of Boxing Postures and Maxims

18 Buddha Hands

Defensive

Offensive

Maxims Continued

Contents

Pictorial of Boxing Postures and Maxims

Back Matter

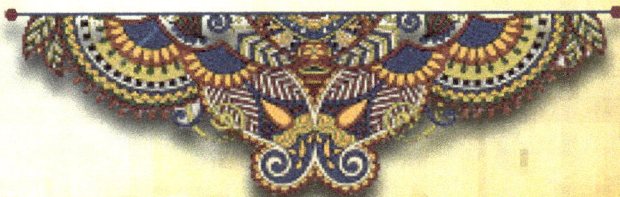

Preface

Some students told me they couldn't conveniently locate these photos and sayings so I decided to create this new edition for easy tote and quick reference. Some of the photos and sayings herein have appeared on my websites or in my books and digital media. This book makes a convenient study guide for the principles, tactics, strategies, and 18 Buddha Hands. The maxims are outlined and listed in the Table of Contents. The book layout includes basic history of temples and lineage.

TRAINING NOTE: In addition to being a useful quick reference, I encourage you to train five minutes daily, each of the senior's Mantis postures shown in this book. Just stand in front of the mirror for 5 minutes and mold your shape into each posture. One posture a day until you have trained them all exactly as you see the Sifu do them, in this book. Stand still five minutes, relax, let the flesh sink off your bones and mold your Mantis shape accordingly. Just five minutes of body posture training a day will improve your Mantis.

I've been living here, in the China Hakka heartland of Southern Praying Mantis, for the last 15 years this visit. I first came to Asia and China some 40 years ago and I'm coming on 60 years old soon. Time flies. I suppose my work in Hakka Mantis is the result of the Som Bo Gin maxim: *Start where you are, use what you have, do what you can*, except with a twist - *go where it is*.

This is my 10th book release on Southern Praying Mantis, in the last three years, and I've just scratched the surface. I do plan to release all the transmissions from the main factions of Kwong-sai and Chu Gar Mantis for the benefit of those who enjoy the training. Most of the factions today are open-minded and no longer see a need to keep the boxing secret. Neither do I.

Some decades ago, I snapped the best photographs of Mantis postures ever. The late Harry Sun Sibok was the subject and we deliberately made two rolls of film, 36 frames each.

Preface

All the fundamental postures were photographed. Afterwards, I parked in a Philadelphia City parking lot to visit Louie Sifu. Someone broke the windows out of the car and stole the camera. I didn't care about the camera, but the best photos of Mantis were lost!

I can attest there is much lost of Mantis. Lam Sang Grandteacher had many B/W photos, from the 1950s, of crouching postures and his first generation students. Lam Sigong was in his pajamas and smoking a big cigar while holding a 'cat stance'. These too are lost now.

Baklim Sibok (Uncle) is coming on 80 soon! And Lam Sang (1910-1991) left us some 24 years ago! Jesse Eng Sibok is going strong at 77! Enjoy the transmission in this book and make it your own through continuous daily training!

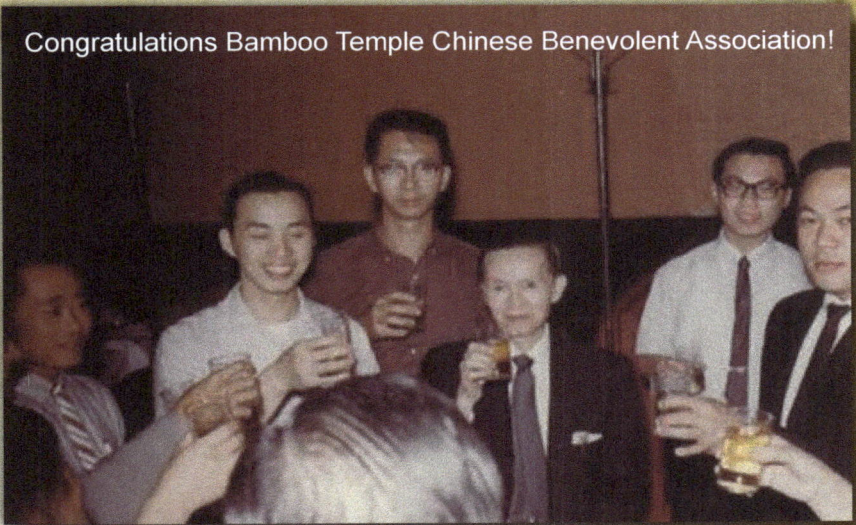

Congratulations Bamboo Temple Chinese Benevolent Association!

Circa 1963, New York Chinatown. Wong Baklim, big brother of the first generation, smiling and happy (left in white shirt) and Lam Sang center (coat and tie). Chen Ho Dun, big brother of second generation disciples, far right.

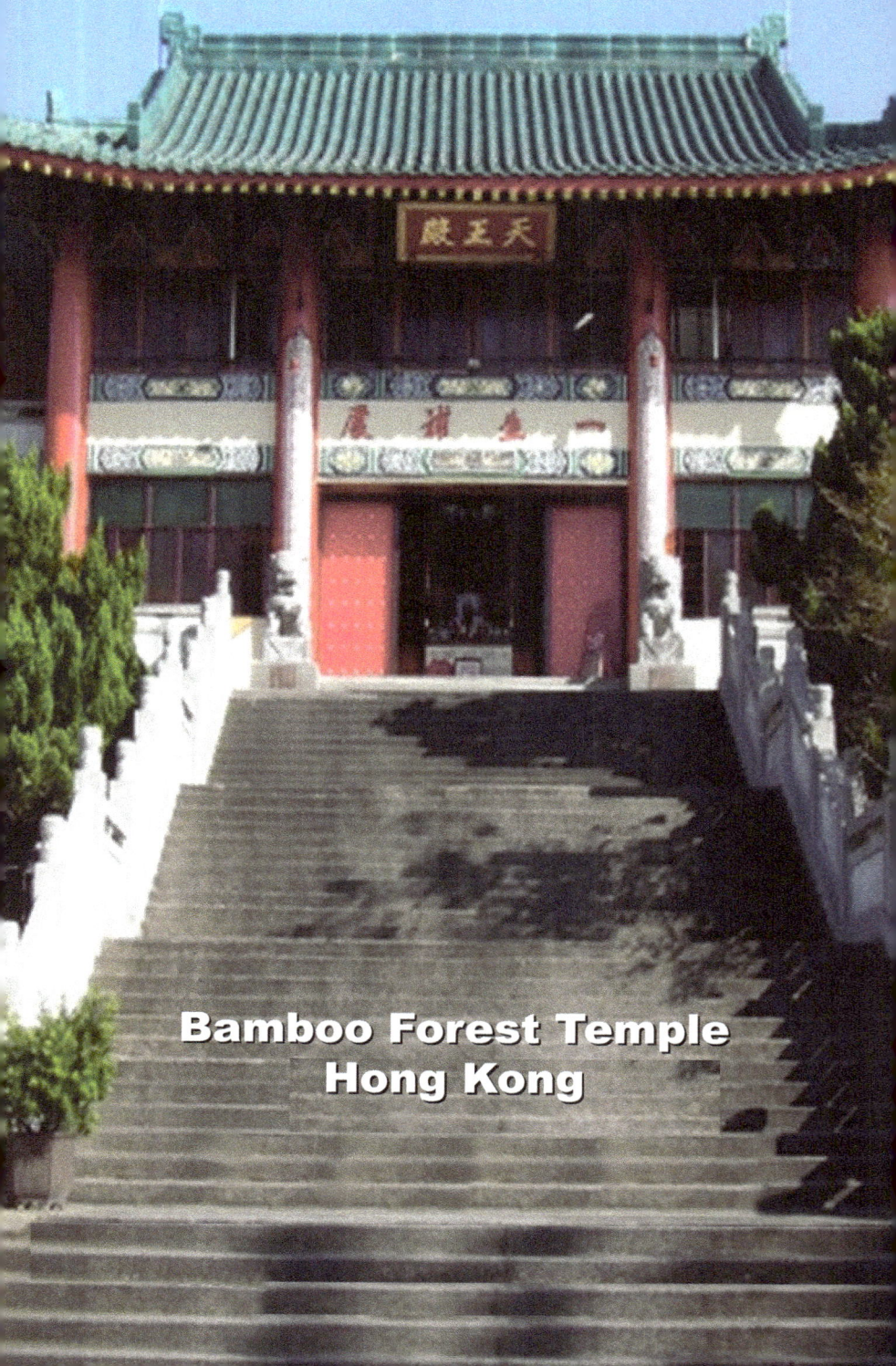

天王殿

一塵不染

Bamboo Forest Temple
Hong Kong

FOUR JOOK LUM (BAMBOO FOREST) TEMPLES IN HAKKA MANTIS HISTORY

Shanxi Province in North China
WU TAI SHAN - FIVE PEAKS MOUNTAIN
The oldest of the Bamboo Forest Temples
has Ancestor Som Dot's Manuscripts

Kwongsai (Jiangxi) Province
LONGHUSHAN - DRAGON TIGER MOUNTAIN
Once set among the splendor of the
Taoist Pope's palaces: Jook Lum Temple
non-existent today

Hong Kong, New Territories
JOOK LUM TEMPLE, TSUEN WAN
A beautiful large complex but without
Som Dot's Shaolin Mantis Order today

Macau, SAR, China
JOOK LUM TEMPLE
Ancestor Lee Siem is 'Patron Saint of Kungfu'

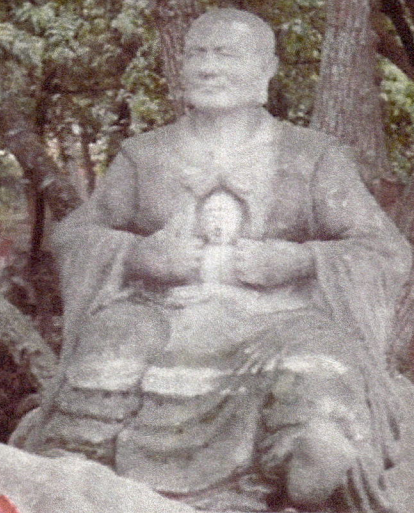

Founder
Monk Som Dot

佛

可圖開父甲寅年秋月吉旦

釋玄倍謹書

Monk
Som Dot

Lee Siem Si   Wong Do Leng

Kwongsai
Mantis   Chu Gar Mantis   Iron Ox
Mantis

Chow Gar Mantis

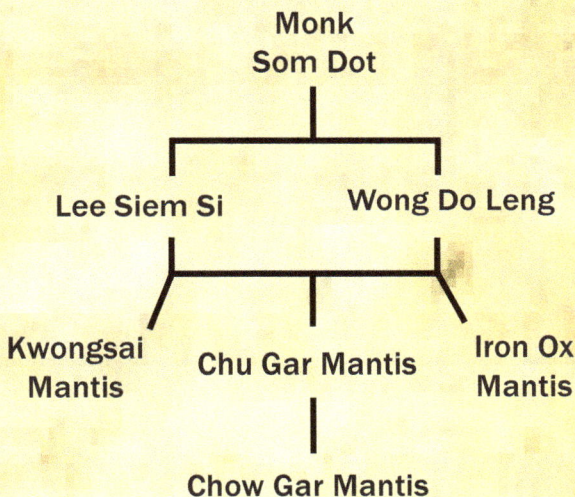

Respect the Ancestors for
their transmission of the art.

Respect the Sifu for his teaching.

Respect the Older Brothers for
their dedication and loyalty.

Respect the Younger Brothers for
determination in training.

WWW.CHINAMANTIS.COM

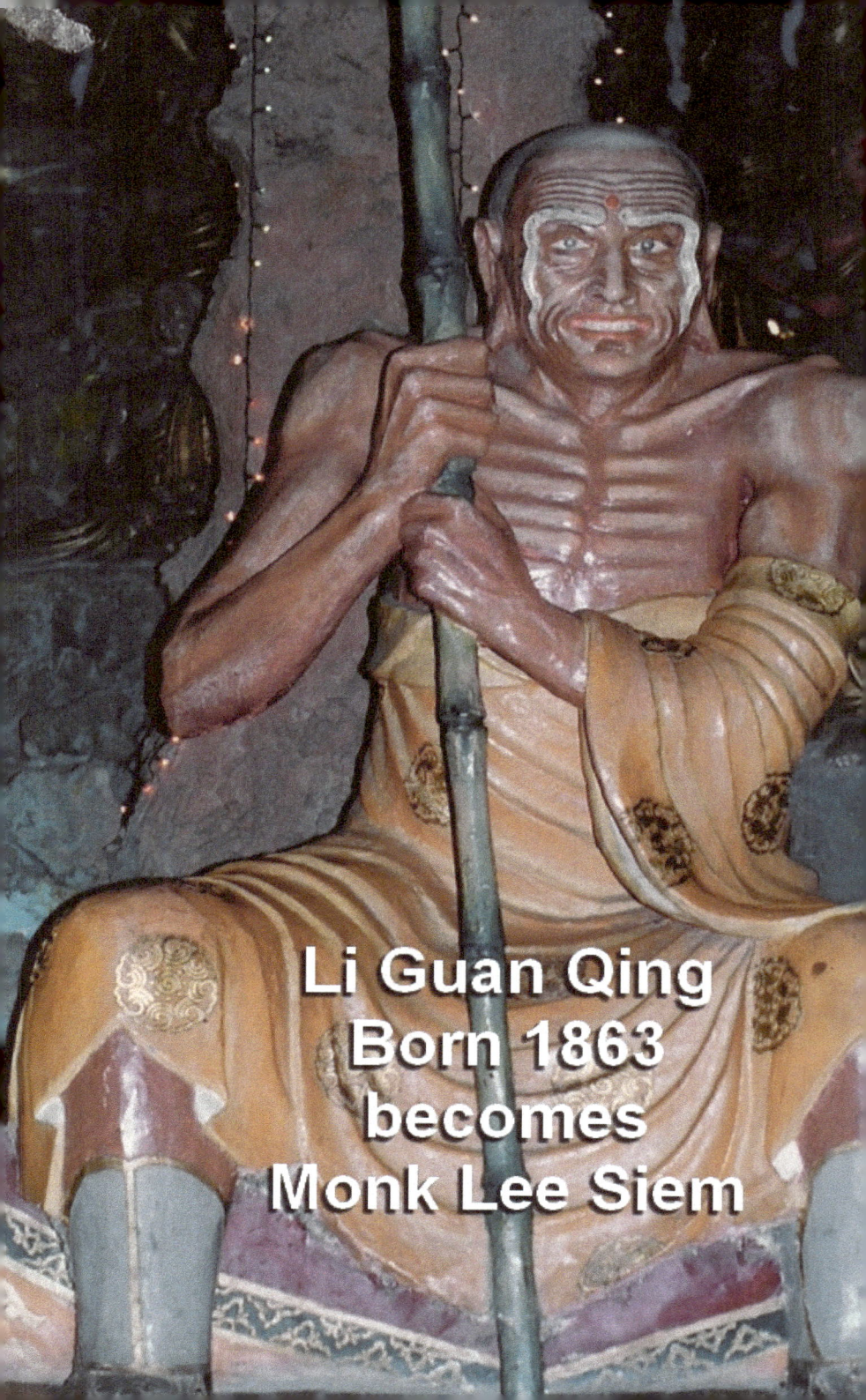

Li Guan Qing
Born 1863
becomes
Monk Lee Siem

Monk
Lee Siem

|

Chung Yel Chong

Lam Sang   Wong Yuk Kong

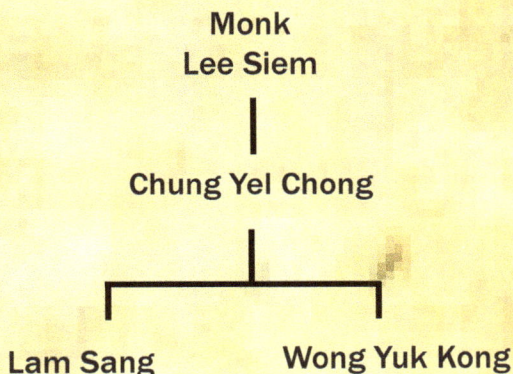

Born as Li Guan Qing, in 1863, the second Ancestor later adopted the Buddhist name, Lee Siem Yuen, which means 'capable of grasping truth'. Li authored several dozen manuscripts using the pen name, Lee Chan Si, or Lee the Buddhist Master. Most of these manuscripts were destroyed in the 1960s by flood.

In 1943, Li's students, Chung Yel Chong and Lam Sang visited Li on his 80th birthday, in the Macau Jook Lum Temple. Li's grave site is said to be located in Taiwan.

LATE GRANDMASTER LAM SANG

(LAM WING FEI)
1910 – 1981

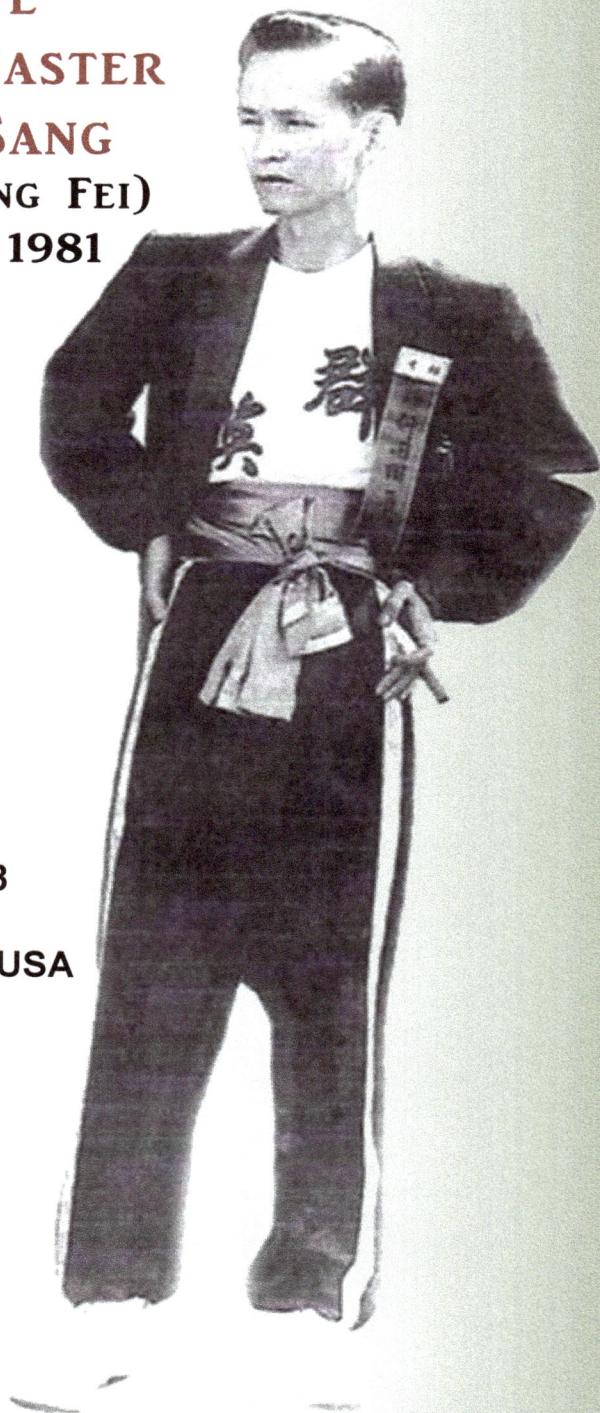

**Image
circa 1958
Seattle,
Washington, USA**

INTENT - WARRIOR SPIRIT

The first principle is intent or will-power.
Intent is simply defined as the
"warrior spirit." Without it, there is no
focus of the body and mind into one
purpose. Strike with the soul, and you
will never miss. Thought and action
are one.

INNER AND OUTER

Inwardly arouse the spirit but
outwardly appear to be calm and at peace.

BROKEN AND CONSTANT

The spring power is broken into
three but the warrior intent is constant.

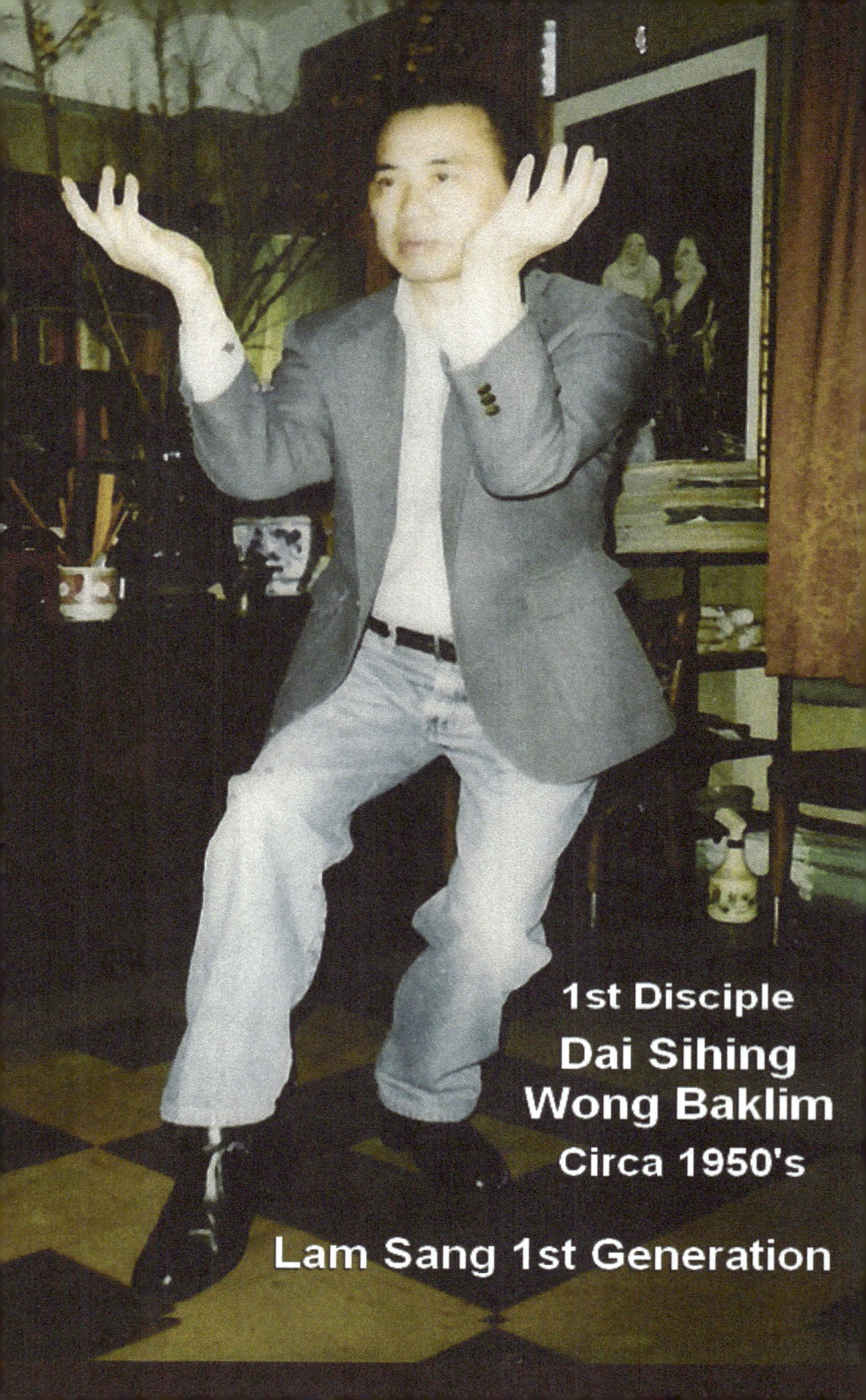

1st Disciple
**Dai Sihing
Wong Baklim**
Circa 1950's

Lam Sang 1st Generation

ROOTING

Rooting is the skill of developing the force of
one thousand pounds in the feet. With it, the
stance is as firm as Mt. Tai and
not easily moved.

Without rooting, the power of the fist will be
stagnated in the chest and one's feet
will not be steady allowing
him to be easily thrown about.

Strong legs and loose shoulders and the chi
will sink down. The root will be deep and iron
steps firm and steady. If one cannot stick and
neutralize after years of training, he will always
be controlled by his opponent.

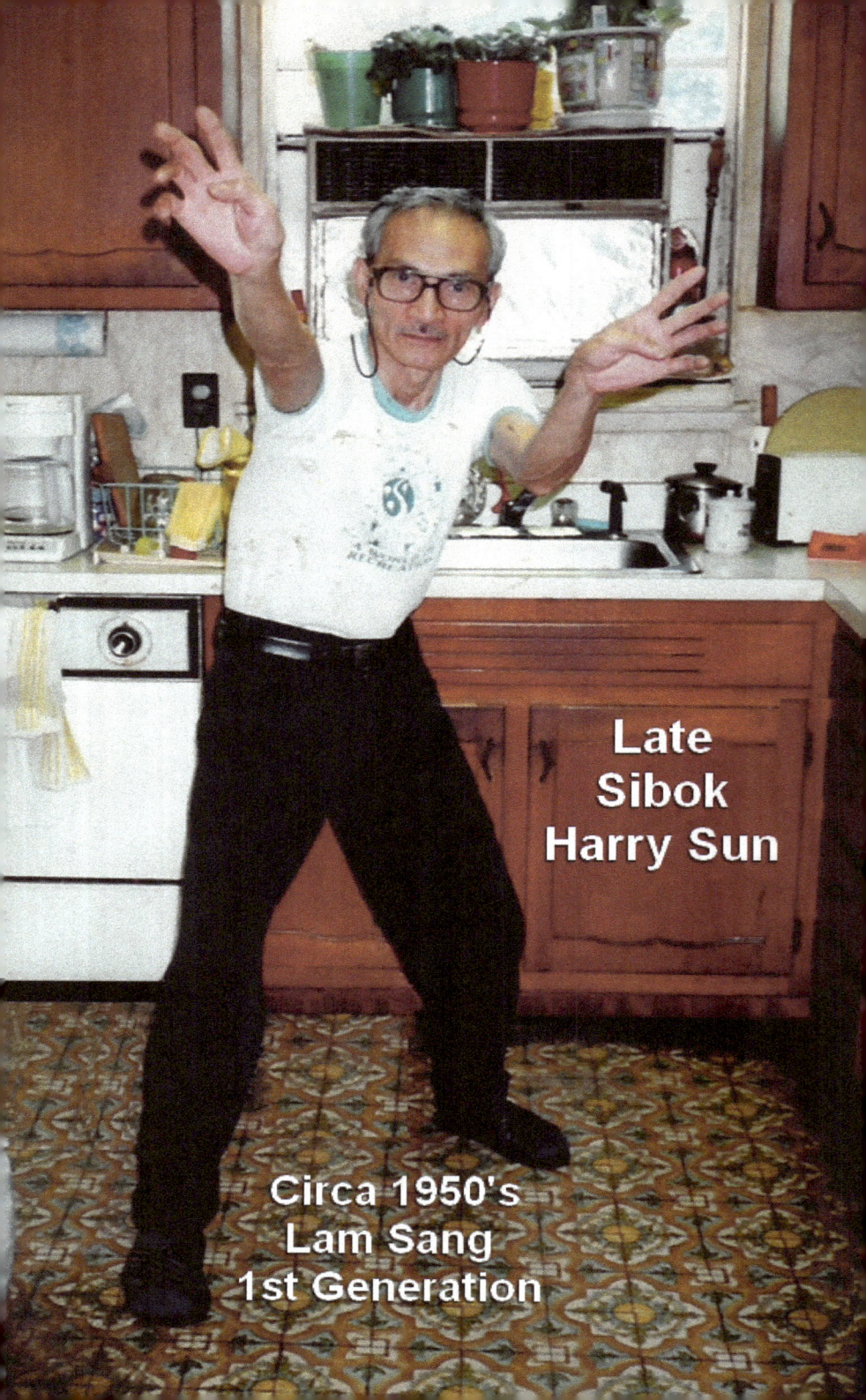

Late
Sibok
Harry Sun

Circa 1950's
Lam Sang
1st Generation

CENTERING

Centering is the development of the root. It is
the lowering of the center of gravity
within the body.

It is accomplished by breathing and correct
body structure. Like a triangle, one must
develop a base in relationship
with the other parts.

Sever the opponent's root and center
of gravity so that he can be defeated quickly
and certainly.

One must develop the ability to disrupt the
balance of an opponent by "feeling" where his
or her center of gravity is and exploiting it.

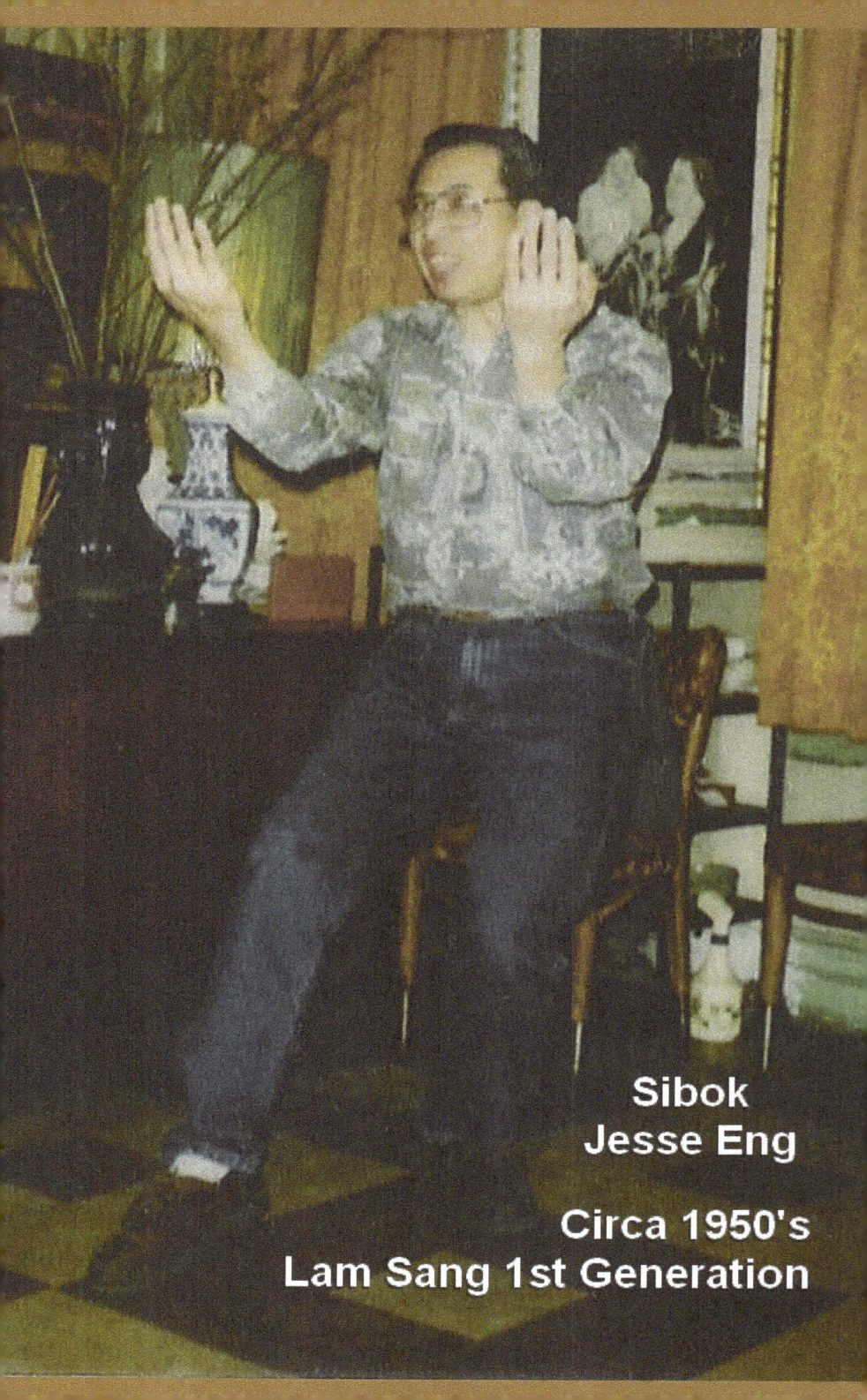

Sibok
Jesse Eng

Circa 1950's
Lam Sang 1st Generation

CENTER AND SINK

Centering is a sinking power. If the stance is too wide, too narrow, too long or too short, the center will be unstable. Imagine an upside down triangle standing on it's tip and you can see the slightest force will cause it to topple. This is a floating center and should be avoided.

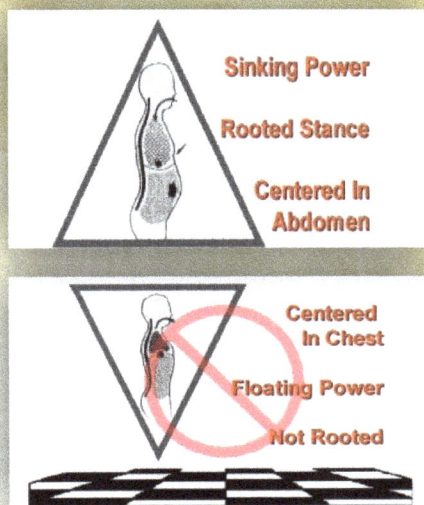

Sinking Power

Rooted Stance

Centered In Abdomen

Centered In Chest

Floating Power

Not Rooted

Kungfu Master Gin Foon Mark

Lam Sang
2nd Generation
Circa 1960's

Mark Sifu's
Promotions have
made Kwongsai
Jook Lum Temple
Mantis Popular
Worldwide!

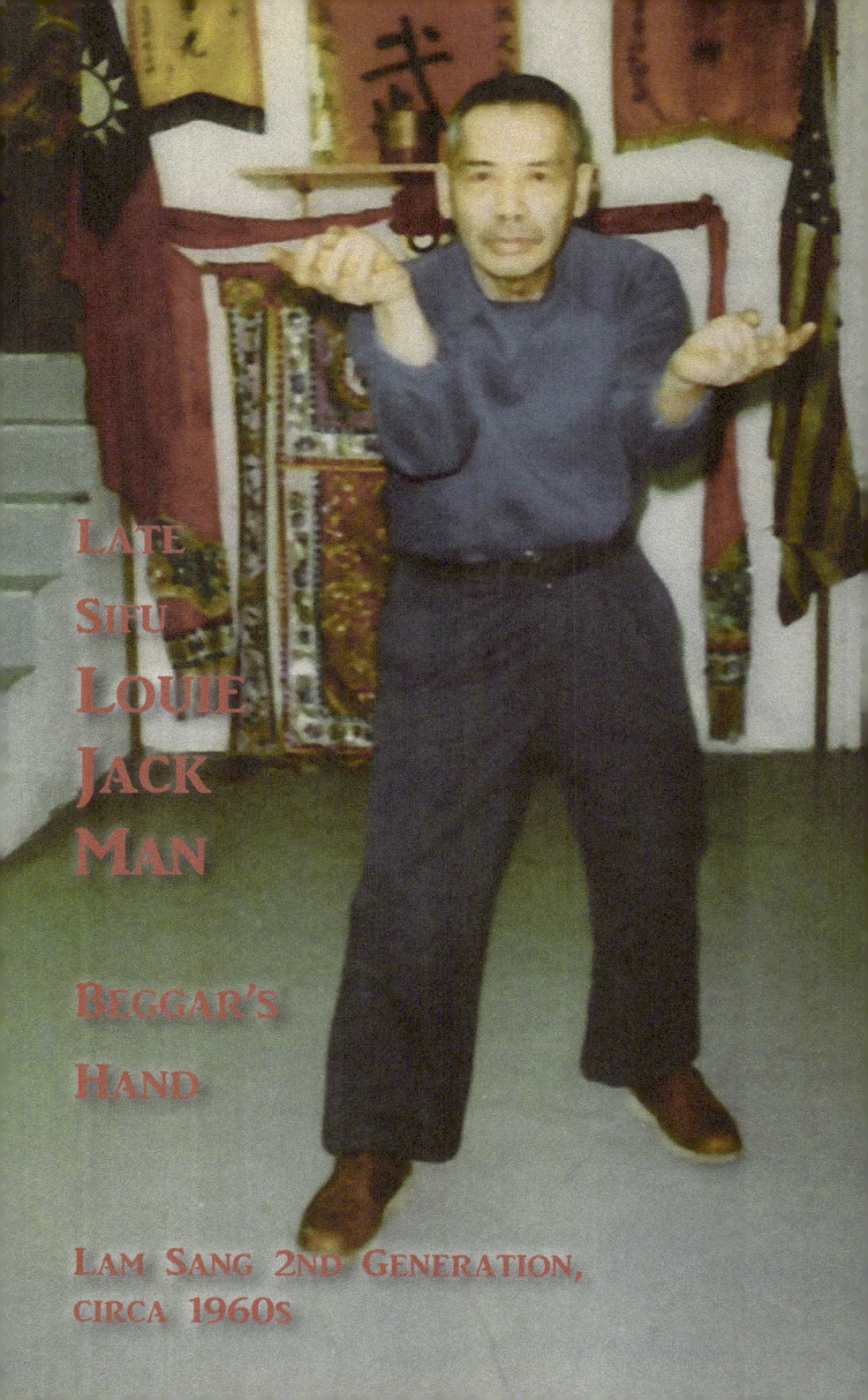

LATE
SIFU
LOUIE
JACK
MAN

BEGGAR'S
HAND

LAM SANG 2ND GENERATION,
CIRCA 1960S

HAKKA MANTIS BODY POSTURE

Eyes to eyes, hand to hand, heart to heart - you don't come - I won't start. You start and I will hit you first and continuously until you bleed.

Hands extended like a beggar, I stand legs like a frog. Heel to toe, centered and shoulder's width apart. Pull up the stomach, push down the ribs, elbows sink to the front.

Practitioners emulate the mantis fighting posture by extending their hands forward, with the elbows slightly bent and tucked in close to protect the centerline - like a mantis. The feet are separated by the distance of about 18-24 inches, shoulder width apart, with the bent lead leg supporting most of the weight, while the slightly curved leg acts as a strut.

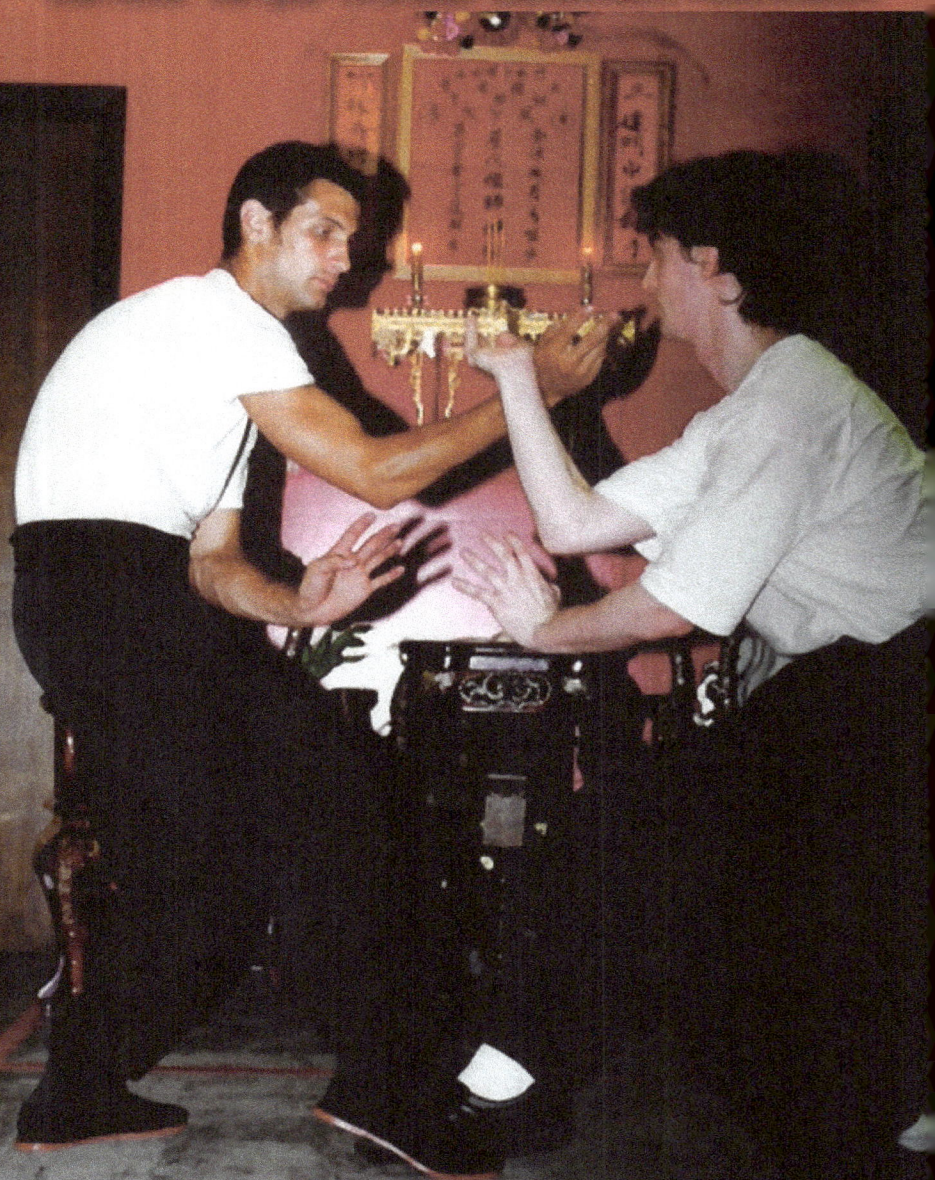

OOK LUM TEMPLE TONG LONG

Bamboo Temple Chinese Benevolent Association

Instructors
Matt Anderson, Michael Feld

SIMILARITY IN STYLES

This style is connected by similarity with the Fukien Crane, Wing Chun, Dragon Shadow, and White Eyebrow styles (as well as the Okinawan Karate styles). Its technique is based on a deep rooted firm upright stance, straight forward explosive force (of a sticky nature) and the use of turning or borrowing power with small deflective angles, circles and hooks.

WHOLE BODY POWER

For the feet, legs, and waist to act together as an integrated whole, to develop whole body power as one hand, one must keep heel to toe and shoulder width apart so that while advancing or withdrawing one can grasp the opportunity of favorable timing and advantageous position.

Bamboo Temple
Chinese Benevolent Association

Join an
International School
or Start a Study
Group Today!

www.bambootemple.com

FORWARD MOMENTUM

The centered rooted posture must be expressed in a slight forward momentum to create a forward driving force in attack. This forward momentum mimics the axis of the earth which is not upright but inclined on an approx. 15 degree inclination.

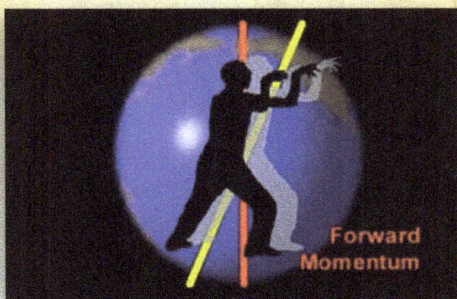

Forward
Momentum

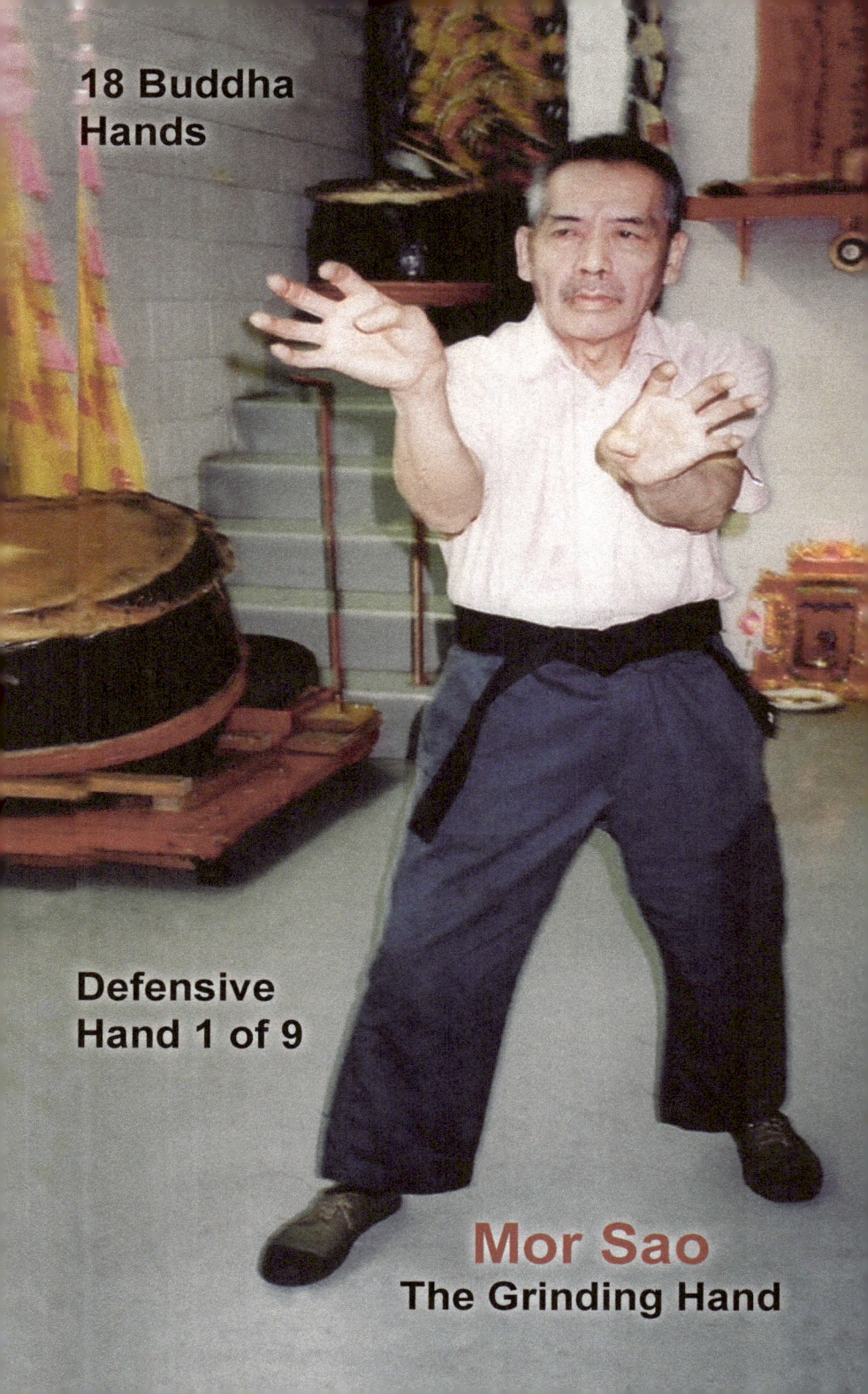

18 Buddha
Hands

Defensive
Hand 1 of 9

Mor Sao
The Grinding Hand

MOR SAO: GRINDING HAND
Mantis Horse is the Foundation of Power

Mor Sao is the Foundation of Mantis Hands
Feeling, Listening, Turning Power
Sticky, Sensitivity, Neutralize

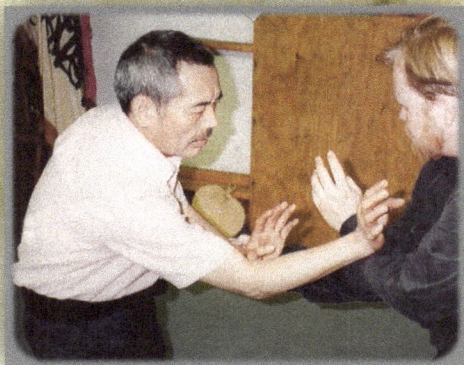

Centerline Defense
Inside - Outside
Low, Middle, High Gate
Single Bridge - Double Bridge

Redirect Force - Slice Don't Bang

Gwak Shu
Sweeping Hand

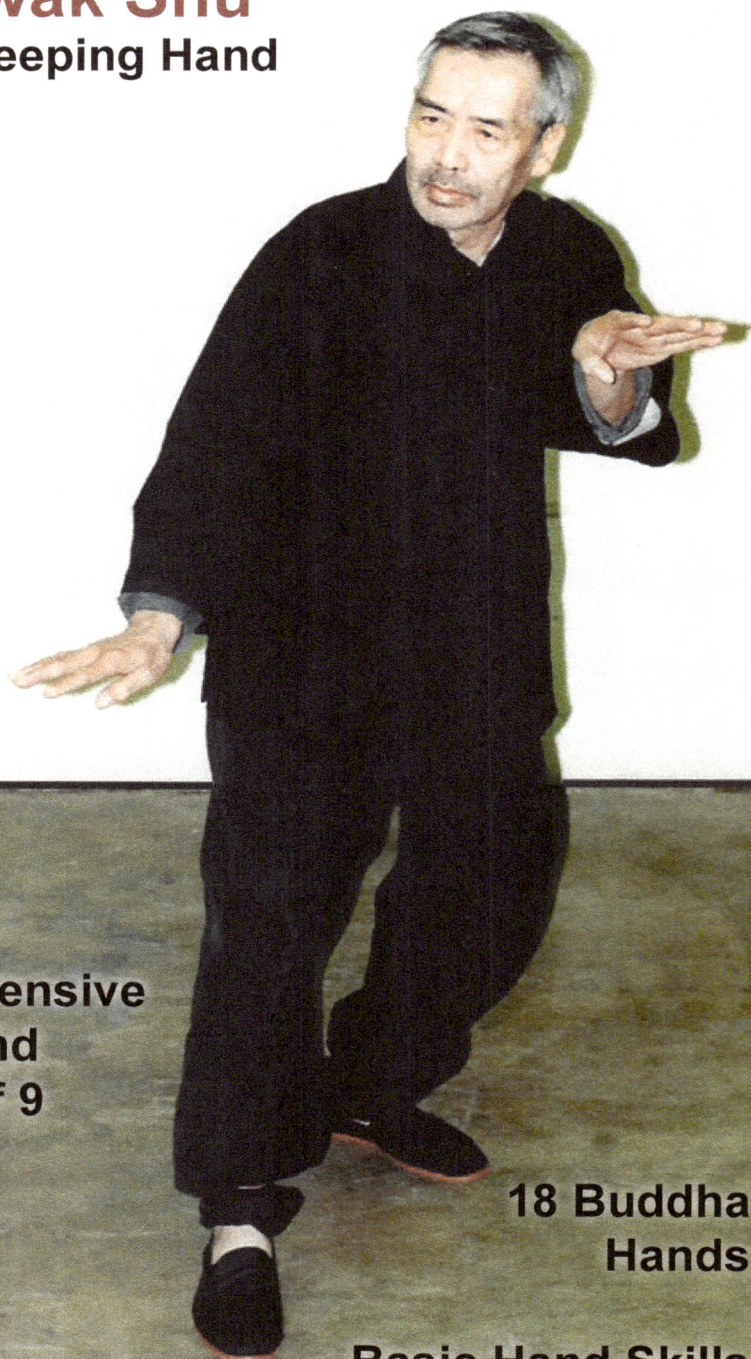

18 Buddha
Hands

Basic Hand Skills

GWAK SHU: SWEEPING HAND
Sweeping Hand, as if sweeping with
a broom. Hooks centerline outward
from solar plexus to lower gate.

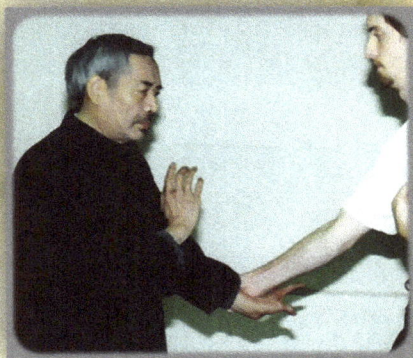

Centerline Defense
Inside - Outside
Low, Middle Gate
Single Bridge - Double Bridge

Mantis Hooks with the Outer Wrist

Choc Shu

Open the Centerline Outward

18 Basic Hands

Defensive Hand 3 of 9

CHOC SHU: OPENING HAND

**Hooks the Centerline outward
from solar plexus to Upper Gate (head).**

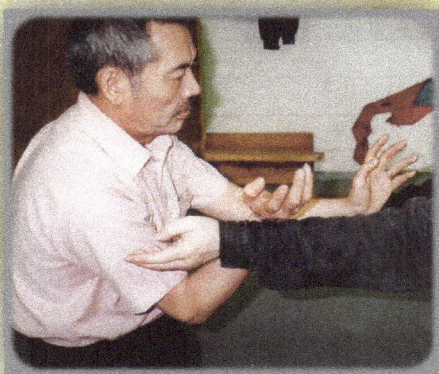

**Centerline Defense
Inside - Outside
Middle - Upper Gate
Single Bridge - Double Bridge**

Mantis Hooks with the Inner Wrist

Sai Shu
Roller Arm

Twisting Forearm Deflection

18 Basic Hands

Defensive Hand 4 of 9

SAI SHU: ROLLER ARM
A twisting slicing forearm deflection
similar to Bong Sao in Wing Chun.
Also used as a simultaneous strike.

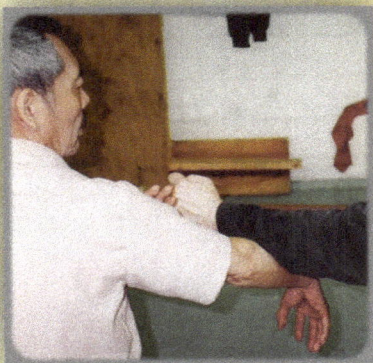

Centerline Defense
Primarily Outside
Low, Middle Gate
Primarily Single Bridge

Slice and Deflect Incoming Force

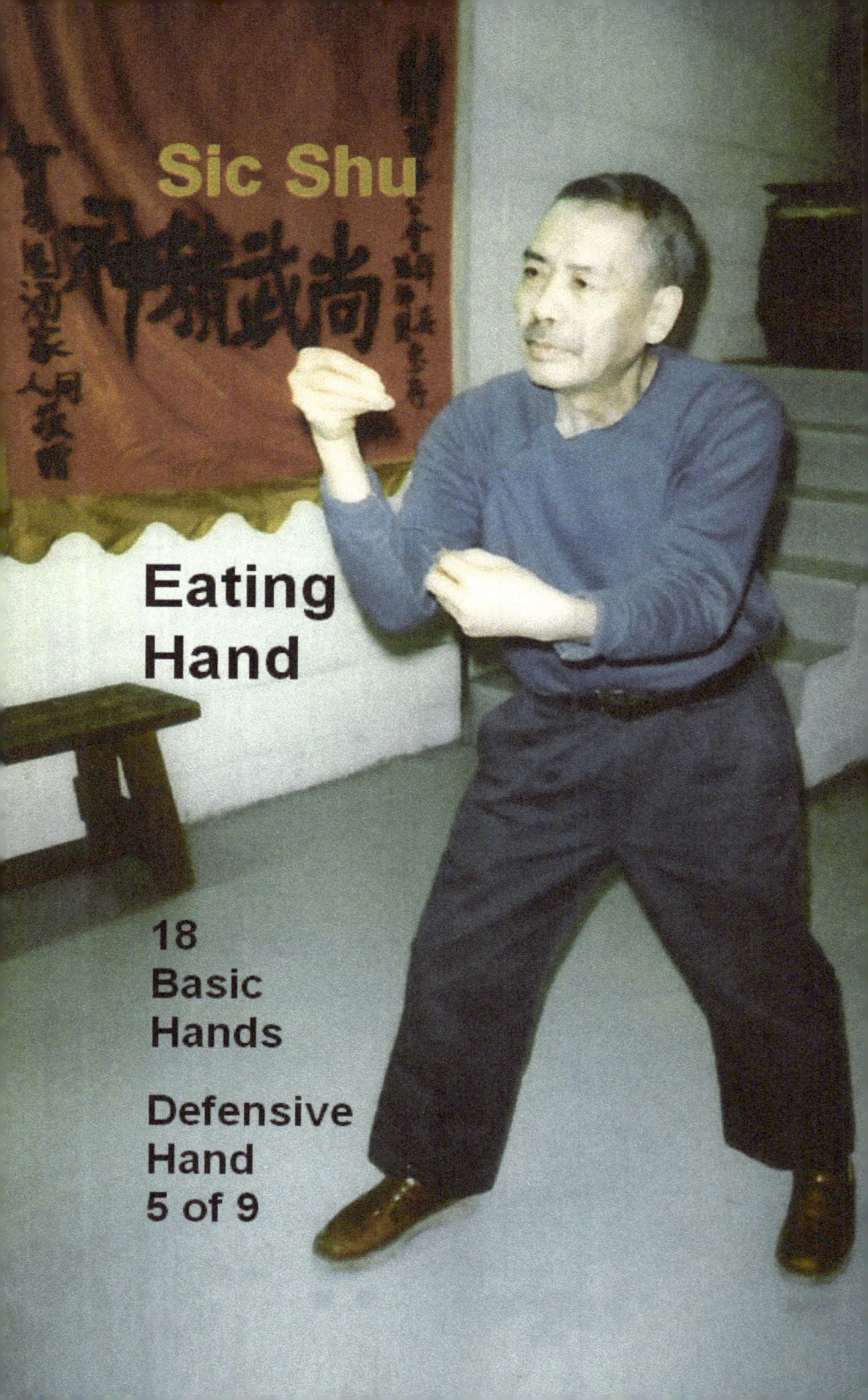

Sic Shu

Eating
Hand

18
Basic
Hands

Defensive
Hand
5 of 9

SIC SHU: EATING HAND

As if bringing to the mouth to eat; Slicing
the forearm across the centerline out
to inside while attacking with fingertips.

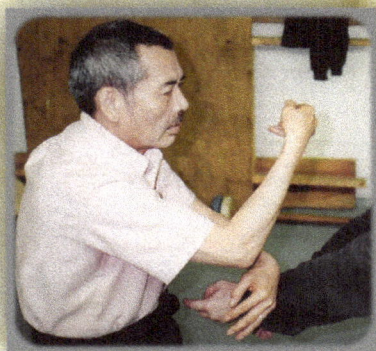

Centerline Defense
Inside - Outside
Middle, Upper Gate
Single Bridge - Double Bridge

Defense and Pluck at Eyes

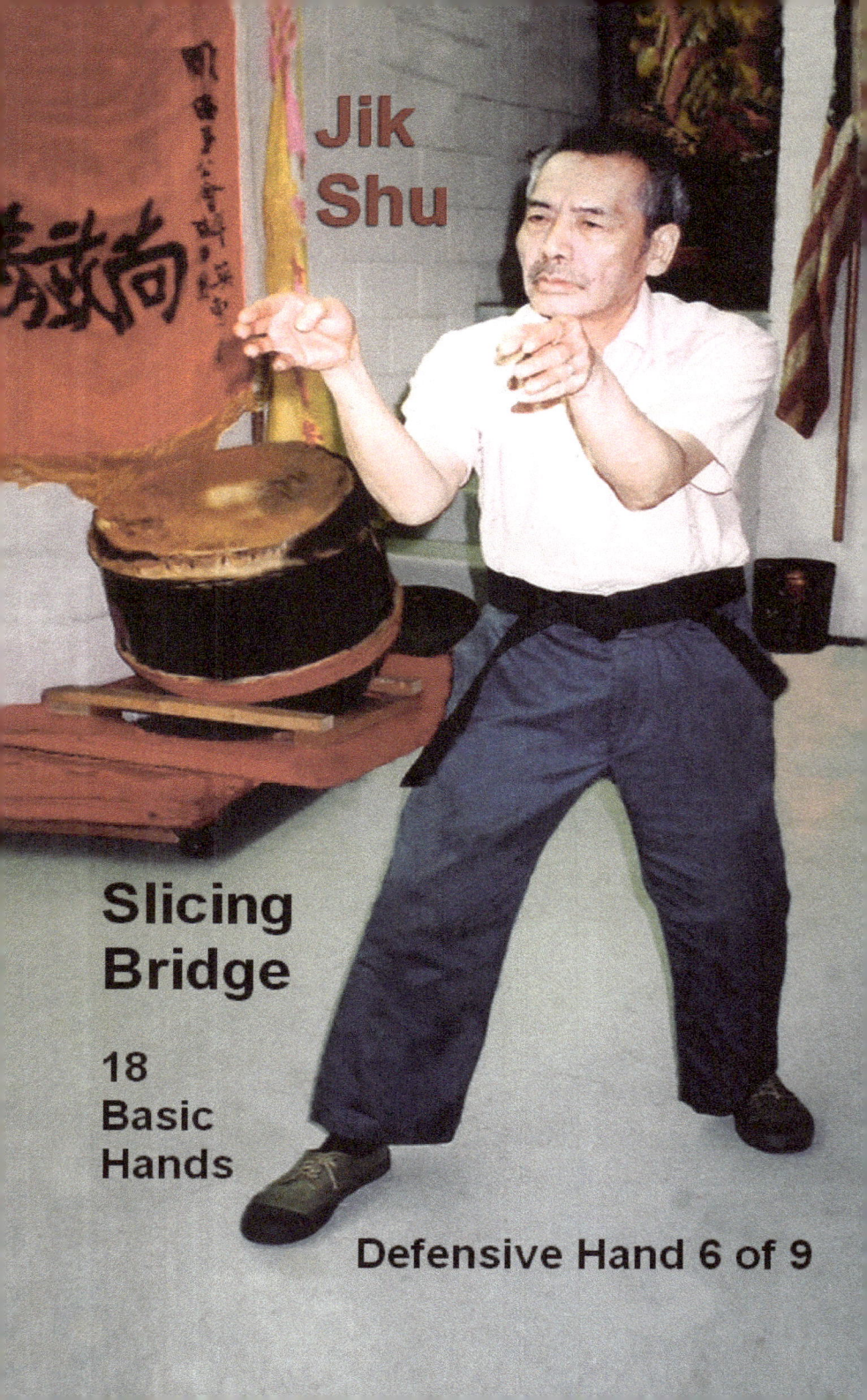

Jik
Shu

Slicing
Bridge

18
Basic
Hands

Defensive Hand 6 of 9

JIK SHU: SLICING HAND
Simultaneous forearm defense (as if an ice skate blade is slicing) over or
under the opponent's attack
with finger strikes.

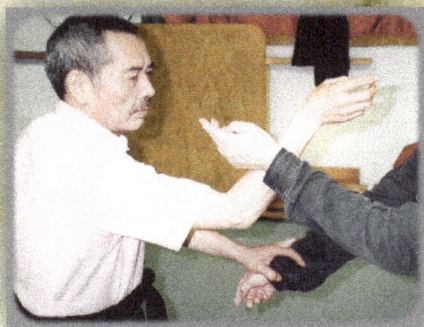

Centerline Defense
Inside - Outside
Middle, Upper Gate
Single Bridge - Double Bridge

Slice Over or Under the Opponent's Bridge

Sao,
Shu,
Shou,
all mean
"Hand"

With
Root
and
Center
the
whole
body
is said
to be a
"hand"

Pak Shu

Palm
Heel
Slap

**Defensive
Hand
7 of 9**

18 Buddha
Hands:
Basic Skills

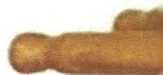

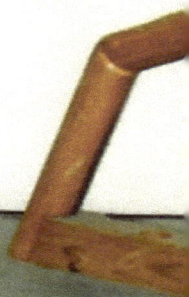

PAK SAO: PALM HEEL SLAP
A palm heel deflection with
spring power (ging).
May also be used to strike.

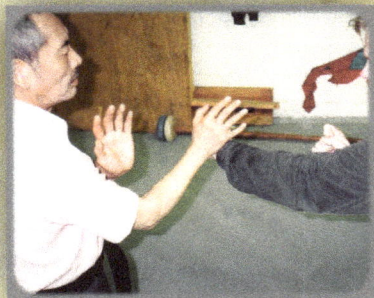

**Centerline Defense
Inside - Outside
Low, Middle, Upper Gate
Single Bridge - Double Bridge**

Used to Hyper-extend the Elbow

Lop Shu

Grabbing
Hand

18
Basic
Hand
Skills

Defensive
Hand 8 of 9

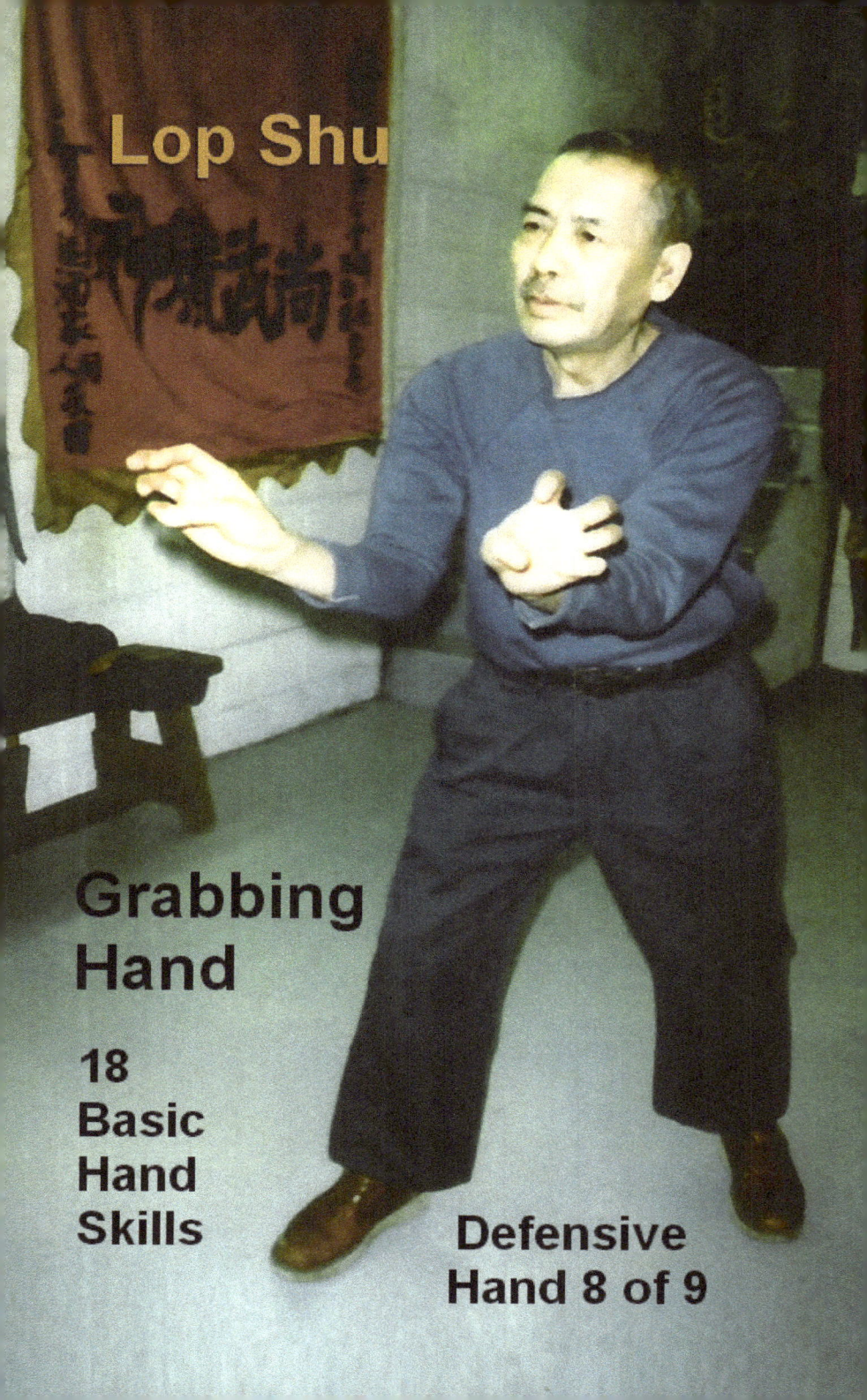

LOP SHU: GRABBING HAND
Basic Mantis Claw to wrists and elbows.
Multiple methods of Qin Na grasping
using the Mantis Claws.

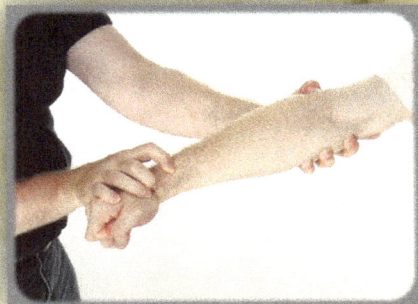

Centerline Defense
Inside - Outside
Low, Upper Gate
Single Bridge - Double Bridge

Multiple Mantis Qin Na Claws

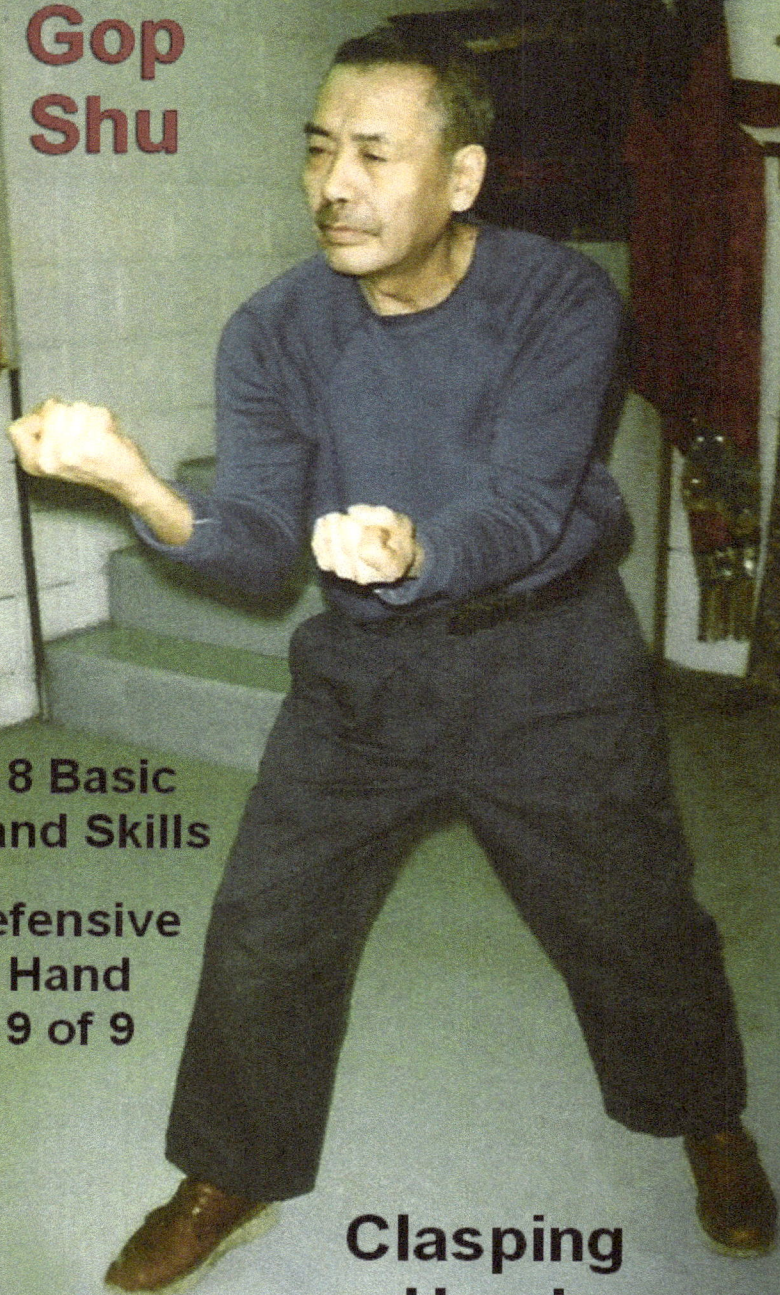

Gop
Shu

18 Basic
Hand Skills

Defensive
Hand
9 of 9

Clasping
Hand

GOP SHU: CLASPING HAND

Capturing and closing the forearms
in a clasp or vice followed by
short power strikes (duan ging).

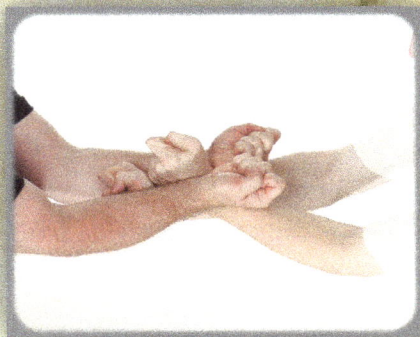

Centerline Defense
Inside - Outside
Middle, Upper Gate
Single Bridge - Double Bridge

Basic to Mantis Trapping

Jek Shu

Straight
Phoenix
Eye
Punch

18 Budhha Hands

JEK SHU: STRAIGHT PHOENIX EYE PUNCH

**Straight punch chambered
on the heart; forearms and elbows
protect the centerline and torso.**

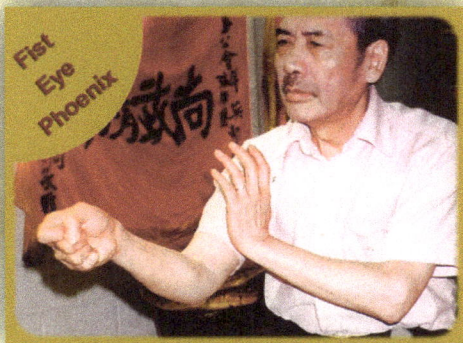

Fist Eye Phoenix

The shortest distance between two
points is a straight line. Straight
attack, circular defense. Hard
attack, soft defense.

Strike straight at any angle (108).

Bao Zhang

Palm
Strikes

**18
Basic
Hands**

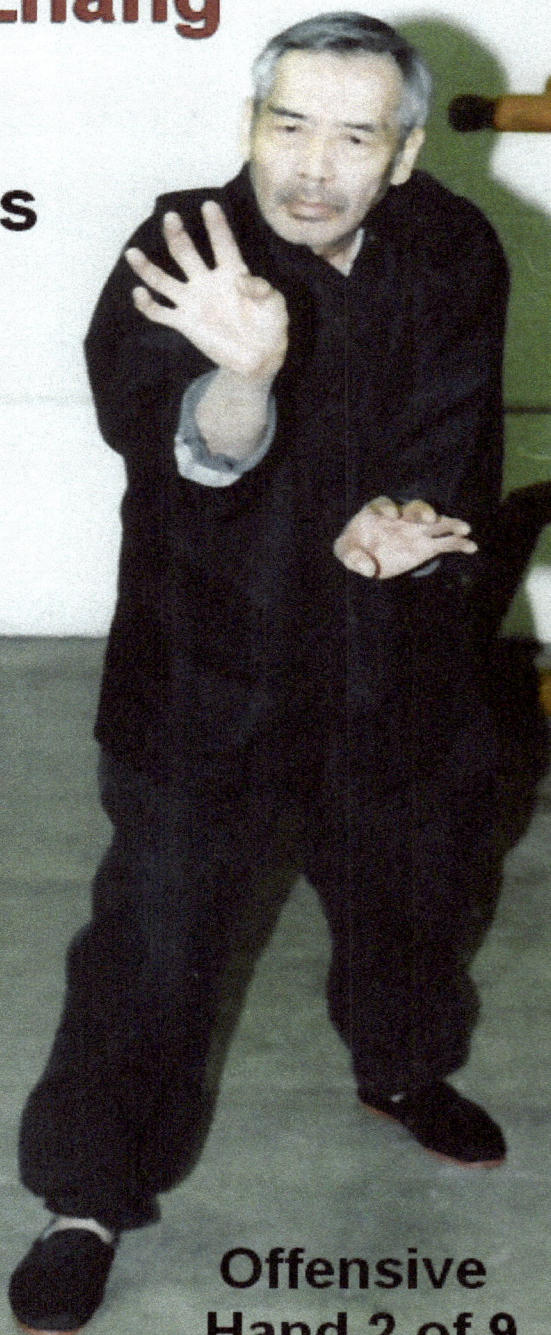

BAO ZHANG: COVERING PALMS

Defense and offense sometimes together.
Cover, bind, protect, defend, shield and palm
strike. Sometimes preceded by fingertip
strikes and then palms.

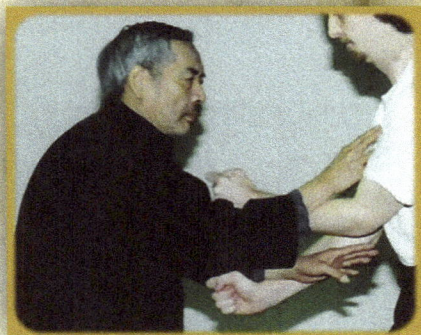

Against soft targets use fists;
Hard targets strike with palms.
Various palm strike methods.

Close the doors and strike with palms.

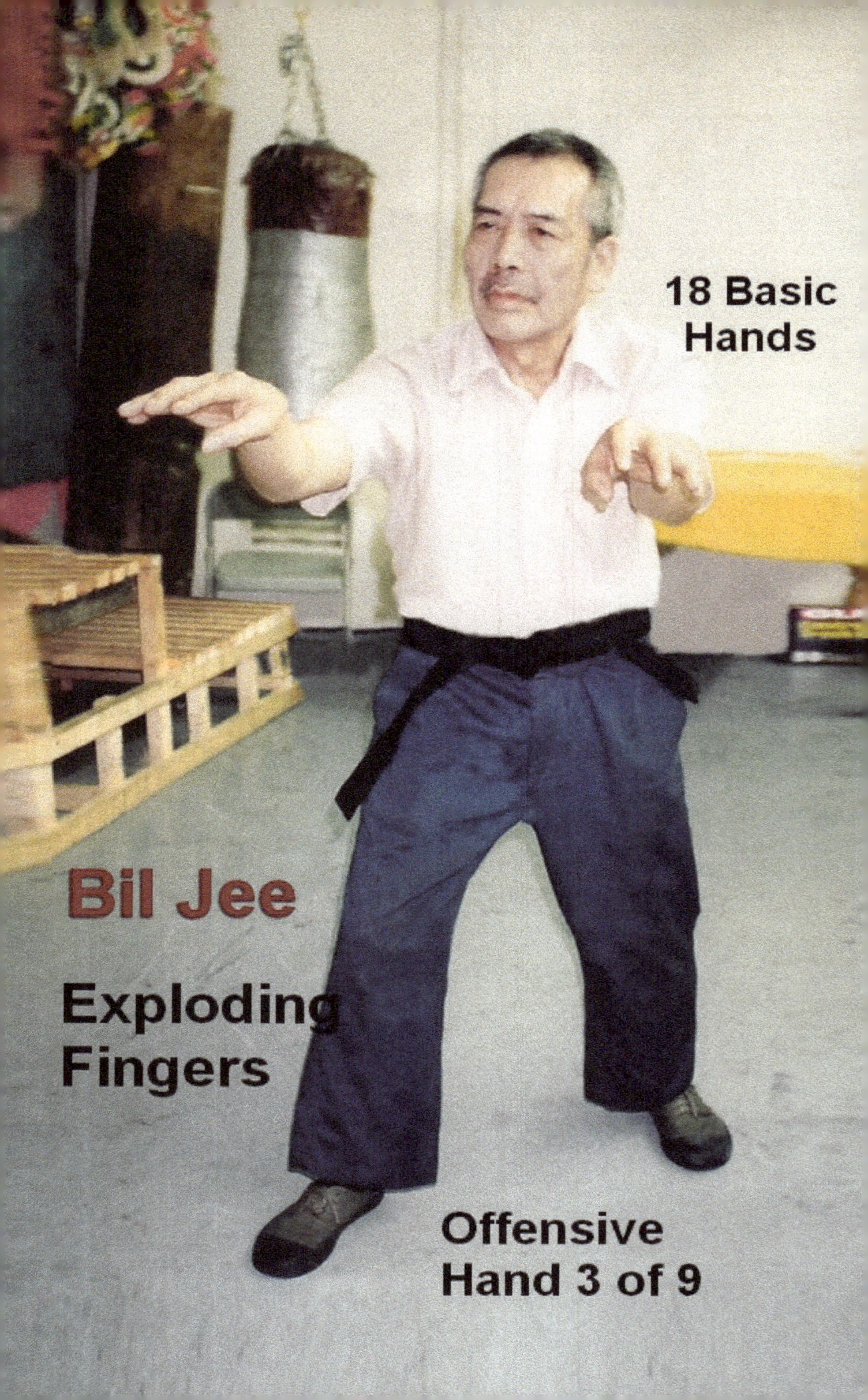
18 Basic Hands
Bil Jee
Exploding Fingers
Offensive Hand 3 of 9

BIL JEE: EXPLODING FINGERS
Crucial Mantis Hand
Many Variations
Fingertip Strikes

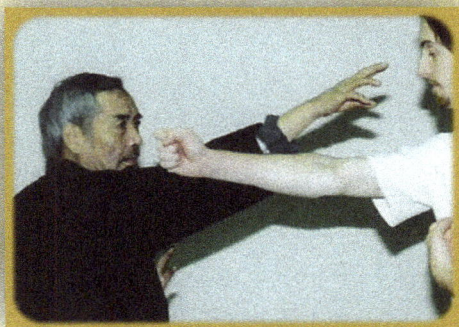

**Grab, Poke, Rake, Slice,
Chop, and Flicking Actions
with Mantis Claws
Simultaneous Defense and Offense**

Standard Hakka Mantis Skill

Ping
Shu

18
Buddha
Hands

Flicking
with
Fingertips

Offensive
Hand 4 of 9

PING SHU: FLICKING HAND
Flicks with fingertips
Strikes with the back of the hands
and flicking fingers to soft targets

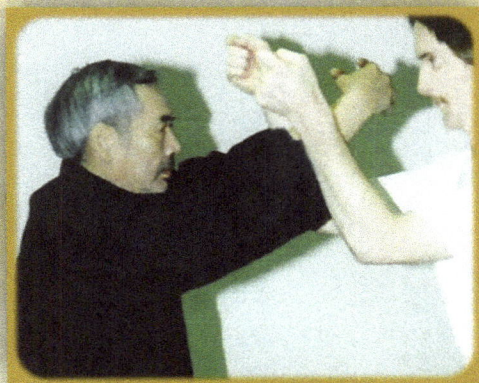

**Strike soft targets -
eyes, inside biceps,
neck, abdomen, groin**

Simultaneous Offense - Defense

Jung
Shu

Uppercuts

18
Basic
Hands

Offensive
Hand 5 of 9

JUNG SHU: UPPERCUTS
Uppercut not unlike Western boxing
Uppercuts with fingers, phoenix fist, dragon fist

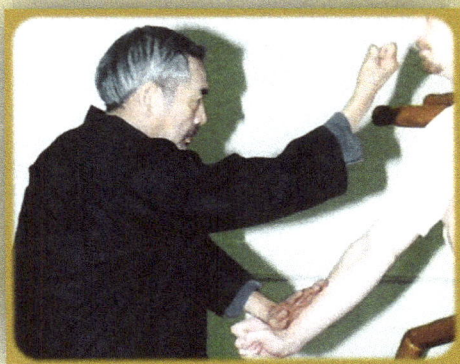

**Like a snake tongue that sneaks
out and over a defending hand
Single Bridge, Double Bridge**

Offensive and Defensive Simultaneously

Chop Shu

Finger
Pokes

18
Basic
Hands

Offensive
Hand 6 of 9

CHOP SHU: POKING FINGERS
One, two, three,
five finger strikes to the
neck, clavicle, carotid artery

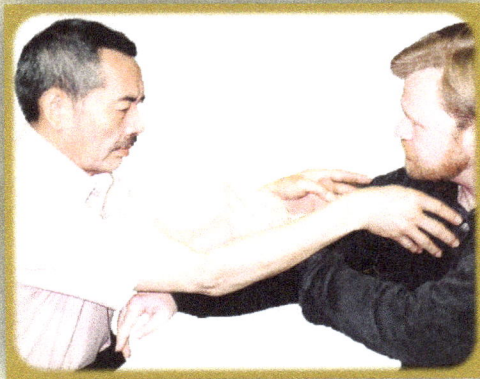

Single Bridge, Double Bridge
Offensive and Defensive Simultaneously

Fingers attack soft tissue

Gow Choy

Hammer
Fist

18
Buddha
Hands

GOW CHOY: HAMMER FISTS

Hammer Fists are employed
after borrowing the opponent's force.

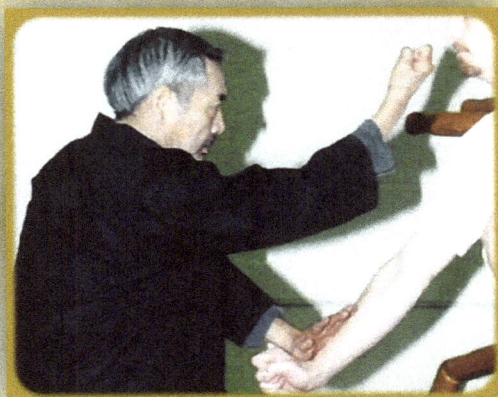

4 Corners and 6 Directions
Small Hammer Fist strikes
Big Hammer Fist Strikes

A key tool of Hakka Mantis

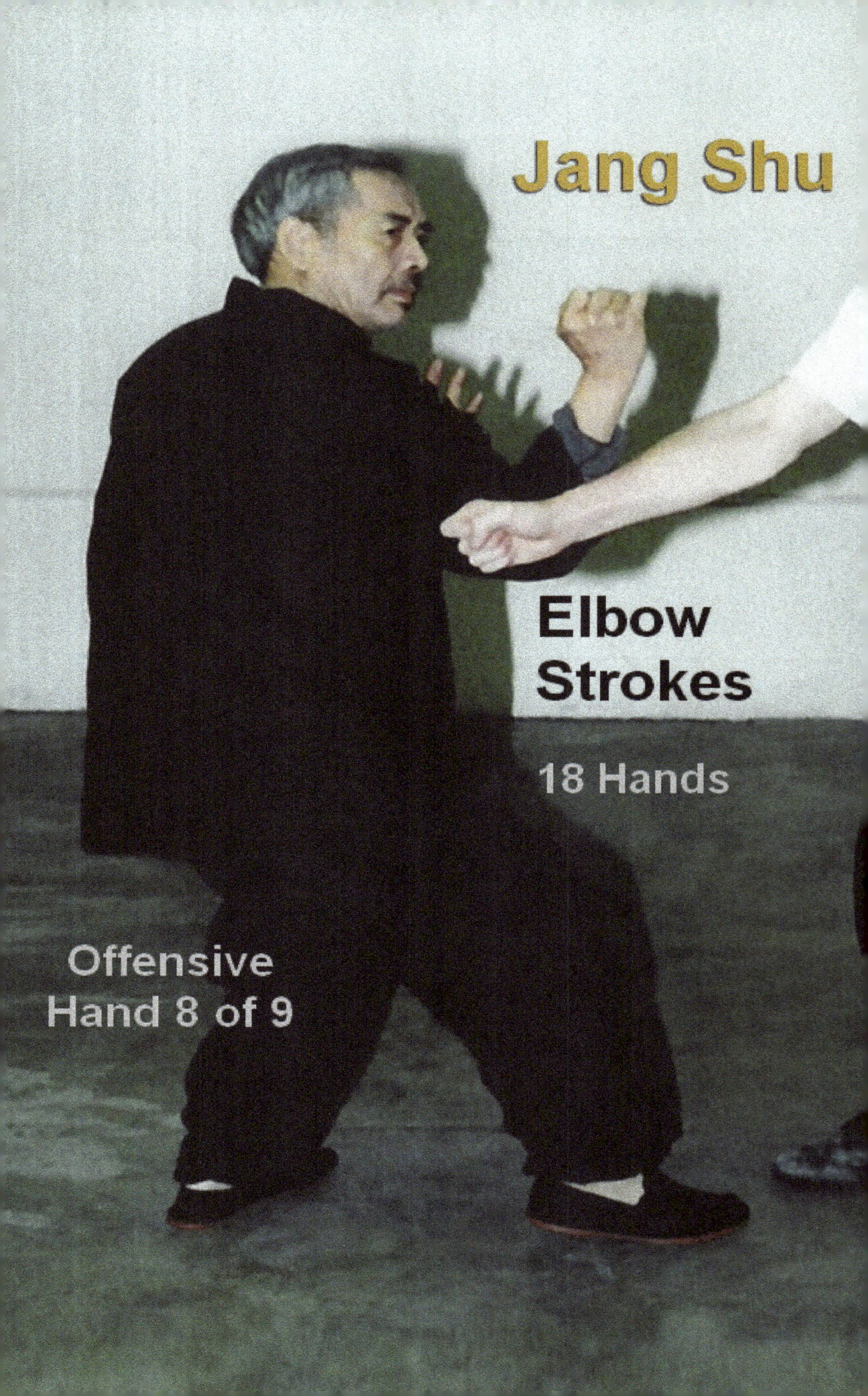
Jang Shu
Elbow
Strokes
18 Hands
Offensive
Hand 8 of 9

JANG SHU: ELBOW STROKES

Sticky elbows are many and varied.
A basic exercise is ten elbow strokes.

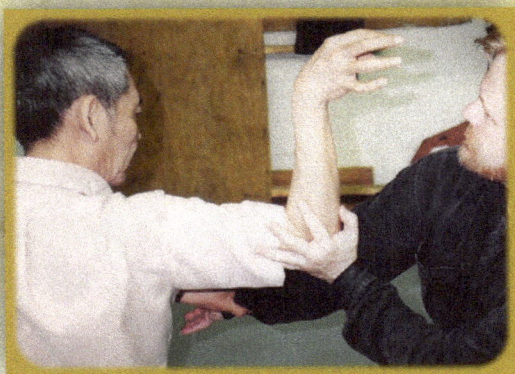

Elbow Strike turns to Finger Tips

2nd Hand Turns to First Hand
One Arm - Three Hands:
Fingertips to Wrists, Wrists to Elbows,
Elbows to Shoulders

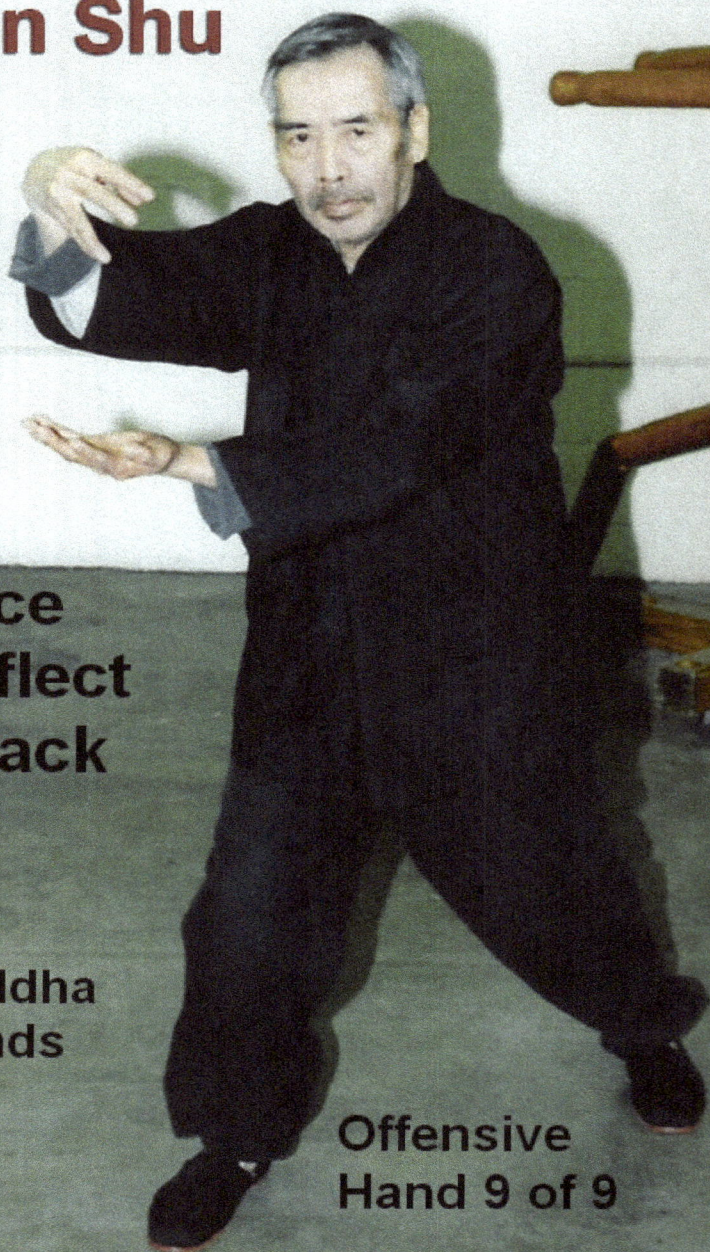

Han Shu

Slice
Deflect
Attack

**18
Buddha
Hands**

HAN SHU: SLICING / ATTACKING

Forearm deflection with a
simultaneous finger attack
and lower Phoenix Eye strike.

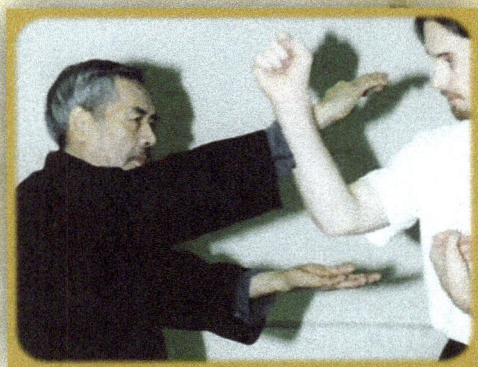

Double Bridge Technique
Enters Opponent's Outside Gate Usually

Lower Phoenix Fist, Fingers or
Palm Attack

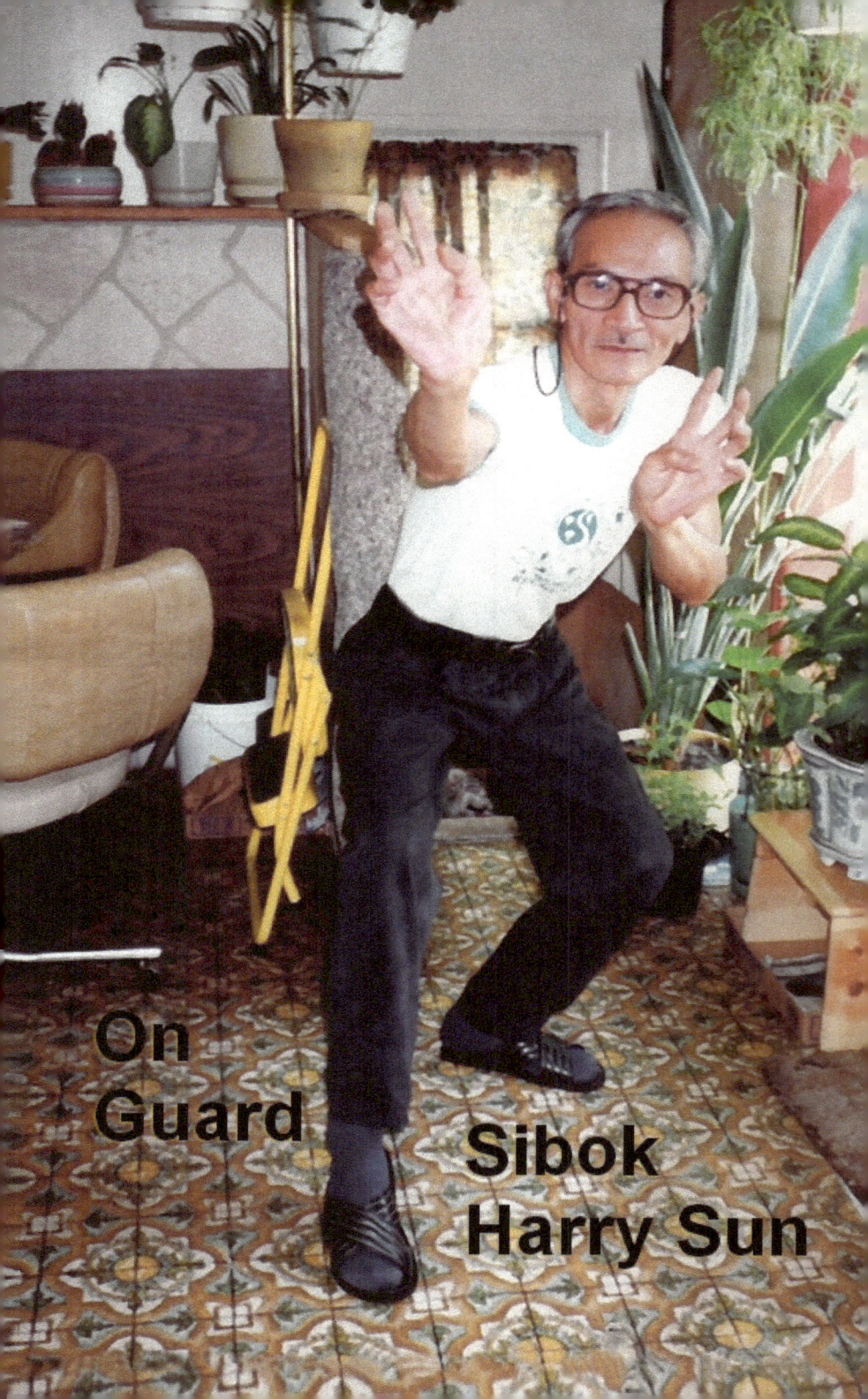

On
Guard

Sibok
Harry Sun

FORM AND FUNCTION

Being that the structure of this kungfu is based on the natural movements of man and the hand movements of a Mantis, the style's form and function express themselves as one.

How many times have we seen dozens of different stylists, all practicing their various forms, only to enter the fighting competition and become indistinguishable from each other?

That is to say, that their form and function is not the same. Jook Lum Mantis is one style that exhibits form and function inseparably.

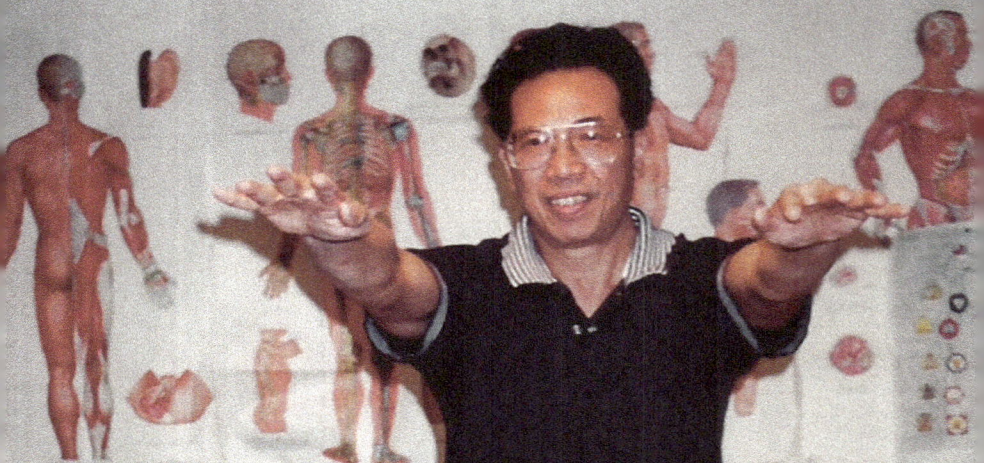

Bil Jee
Exploding
Fingers

Sibok
Jesse
Eng

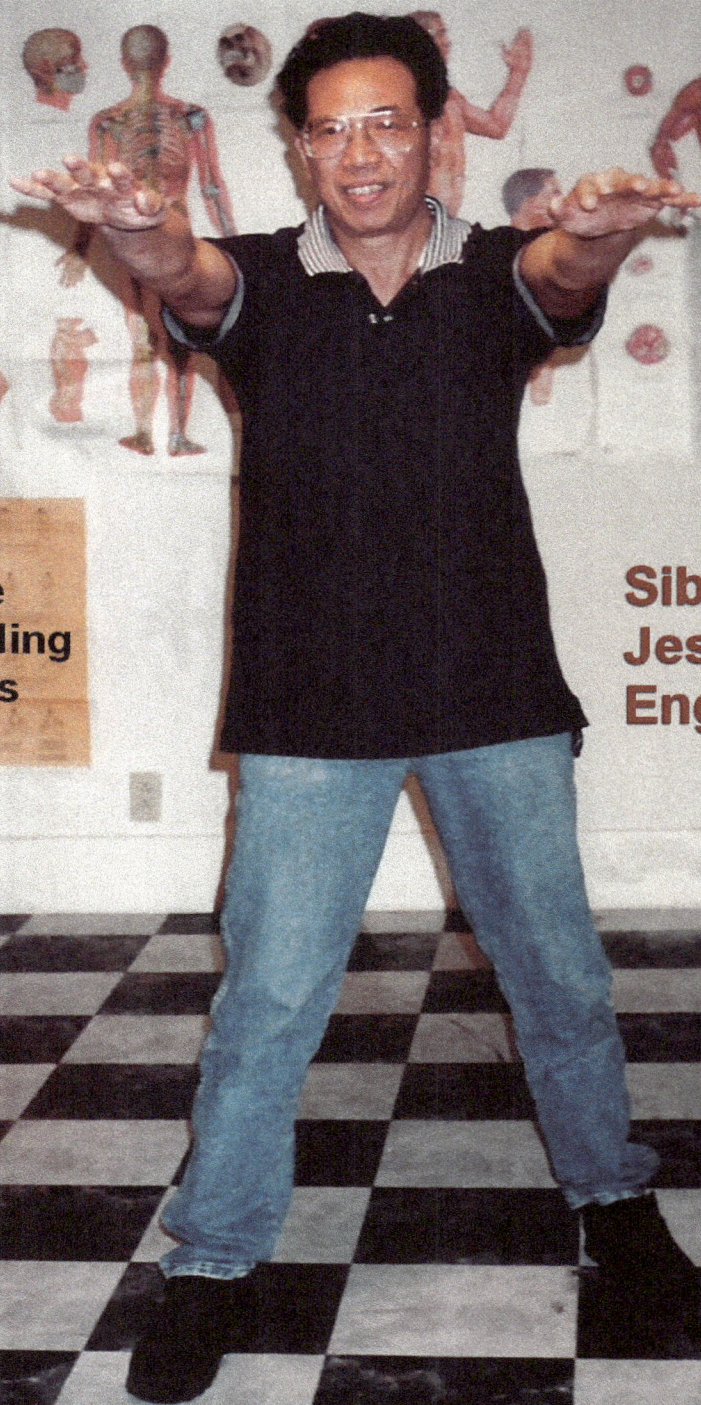

PHYSICAL TRAITS

As in any martial art one must develop
Balance, Timing, Speed, Strength,
and Coordination.

Balance from stance, Timing from not being afraid, Speed from repitition, Strength
from two man live training, Coordination
from self exertion.

Timing is more important than speed.

The hand going out does not miss the
target (timing). The hand coming back
always brings something with it
(off the opponent).

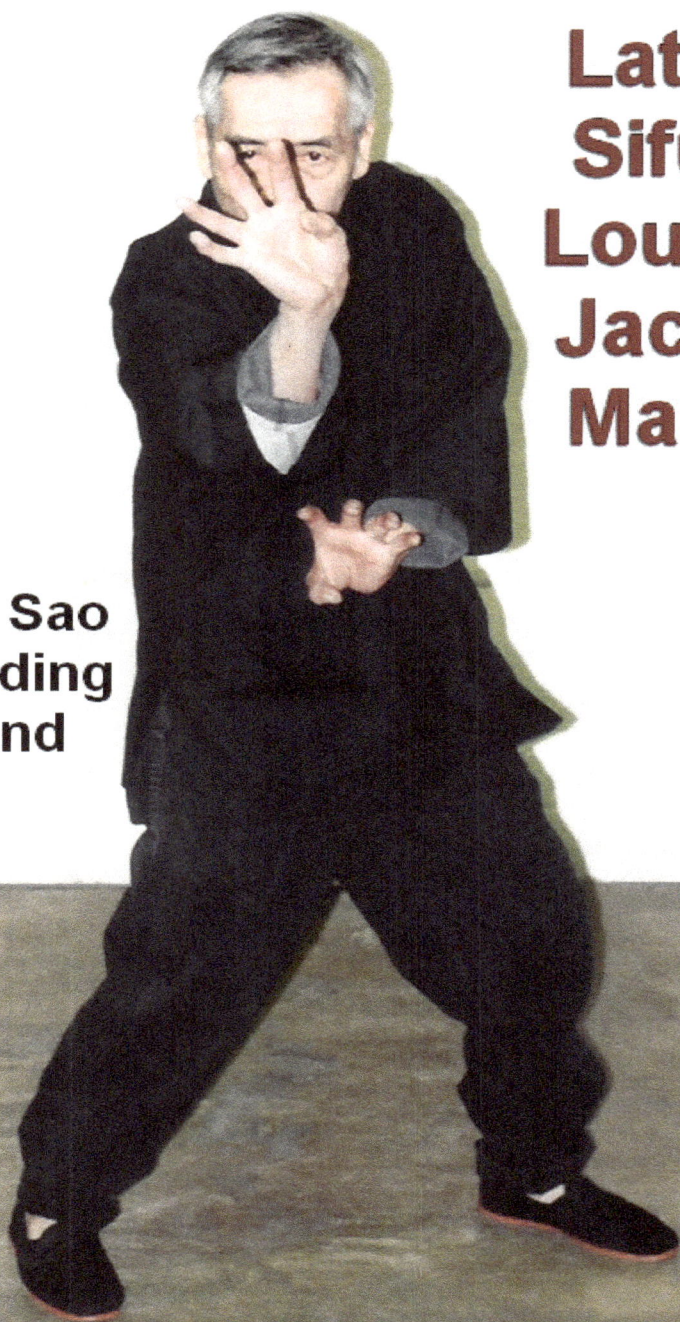

Late
Sifu
Louie
Jack
Man

Mor Sao
Grinding
Hand

BODY WEAPONS

When issuing three power rooted spring force, one may employ various bodily weapons in striking; head, shoulders, elbows, forearms, wrists, fists (back fist, panther, ginger fist, phoenix, dragon, snake, thumb strikes, hammer fist), fingers, palms, hips, knees, shins, ankles, feet, and toes.

1 ARM - 3 HANDS

Defend and attack with one arm is done by using the forearm for defensive movement while simultaneously attacking with the hand or fingers.

This can only be accomplished if one has understood the centerline theory.

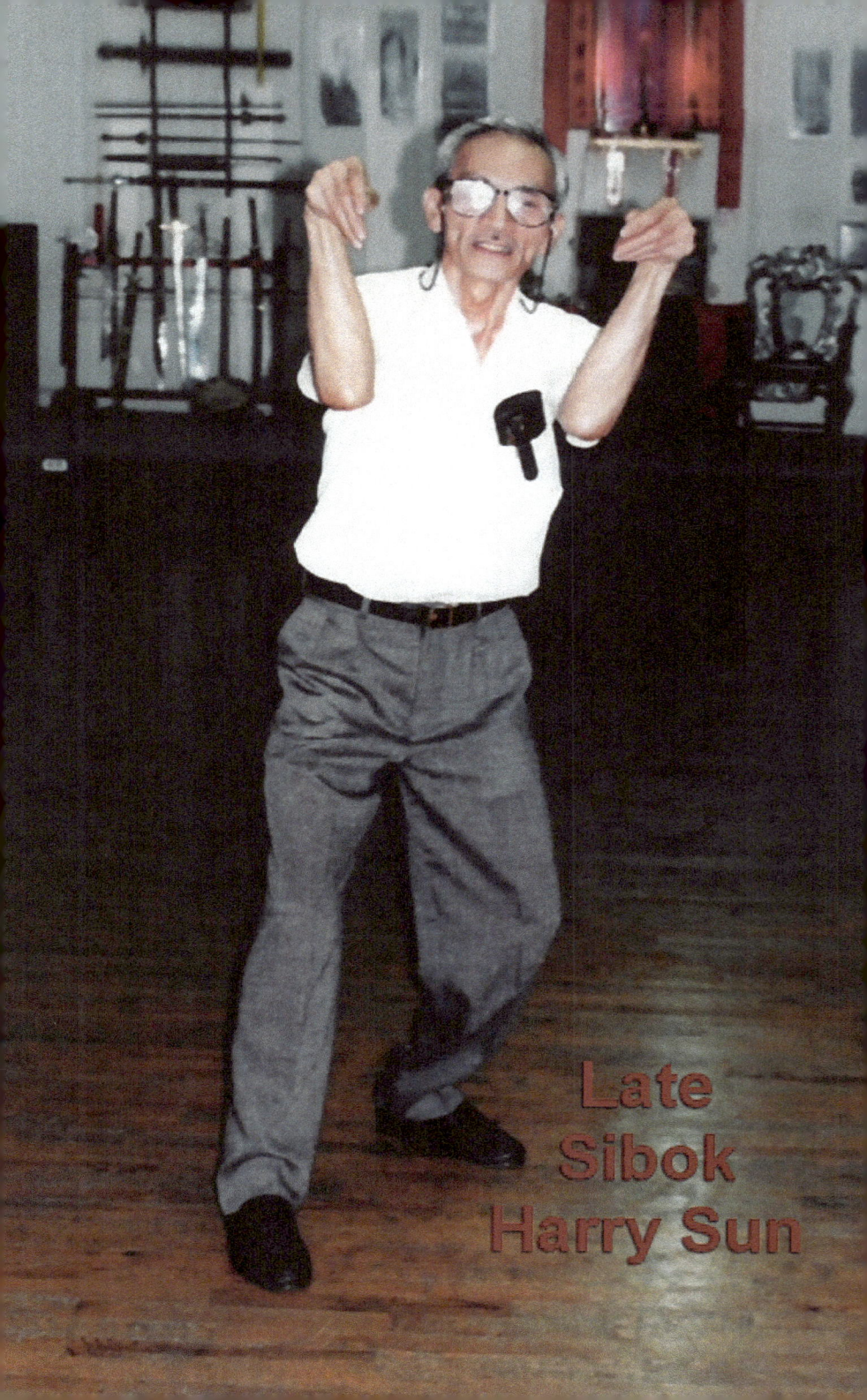

Late
Sibok
Harry Sun

CENTERLINE THEORY

Centerline theory is military science (i.e. pistol training). To stop a man dead in his tracks, destroy the brain; Secondary target, the heart, although the aggressor may continue to live 6 minutes and fight 3 of them. The next weakest links in the chain of life are the internal organs. All these lie on the center line. In mantis, the forearms and elbows are used to protect the centerline.

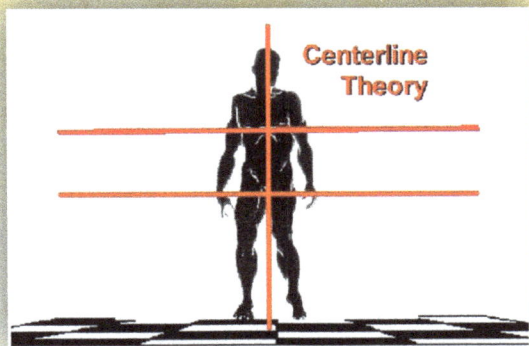

Centerline Theory

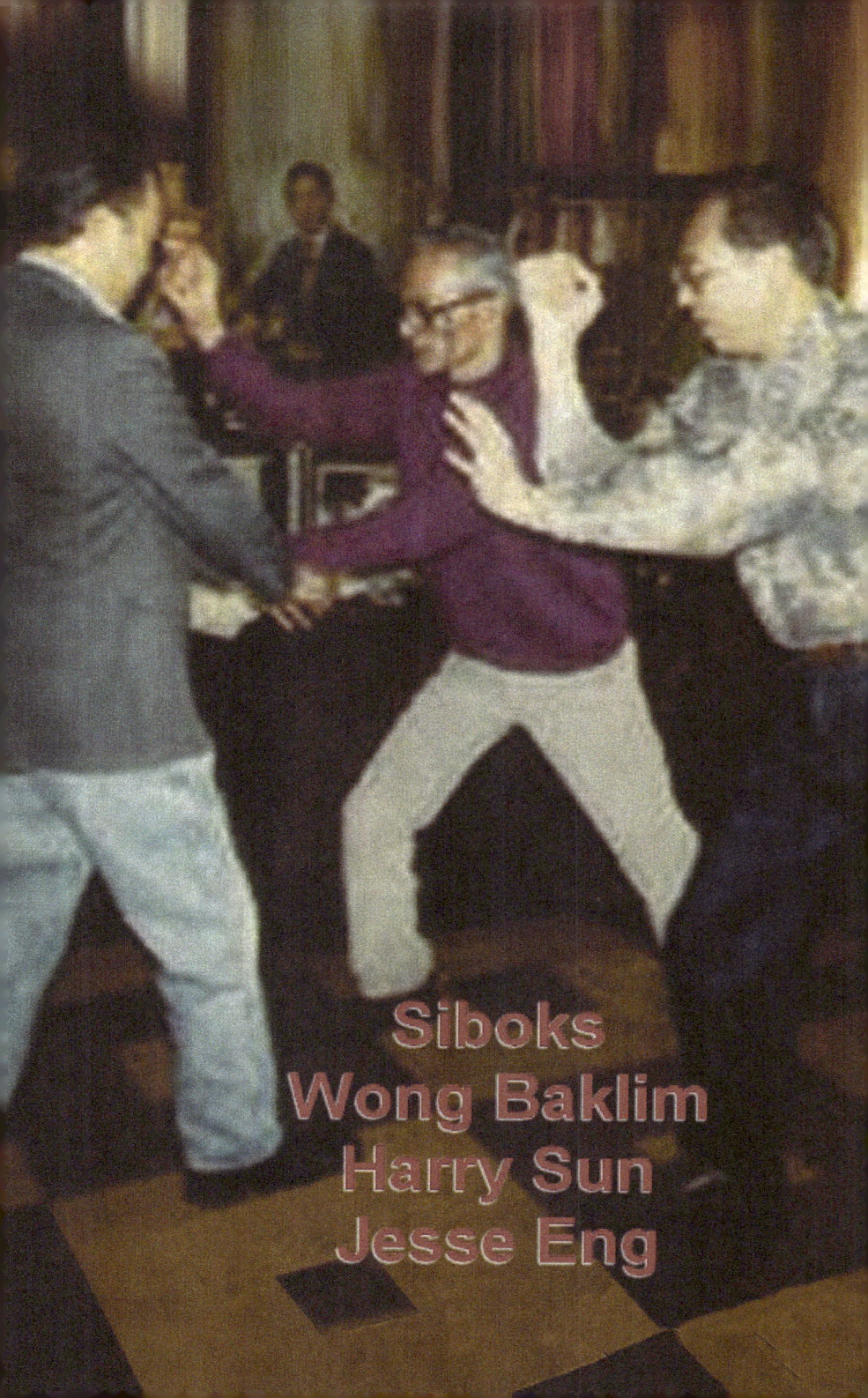

Siboks
Wong Baklim
Harry Sun
Jesse Eng

SPRING POWER

"Mei Hoc Kuen Do, Xin Hoc Ging"
Before you train the boxing, train ging
explosive spring power force.

This produces a live springy power (action-reaction force in a sticky way). It is produced by the whole body in spiraling motions, as a spring is twisted and then released. It is the function of the hand and foot arriving at the target intently at the same time. There is a saying, "any deficiency of power in the hand, can be found in the root and center."

The hand moves, the arm rotates and the weight is transferred from the ground up the heels matching in the ankles, knees and hips.

When rooting, spring and spiral becomes skillful, one feels as if he is anchored fully to the earth.

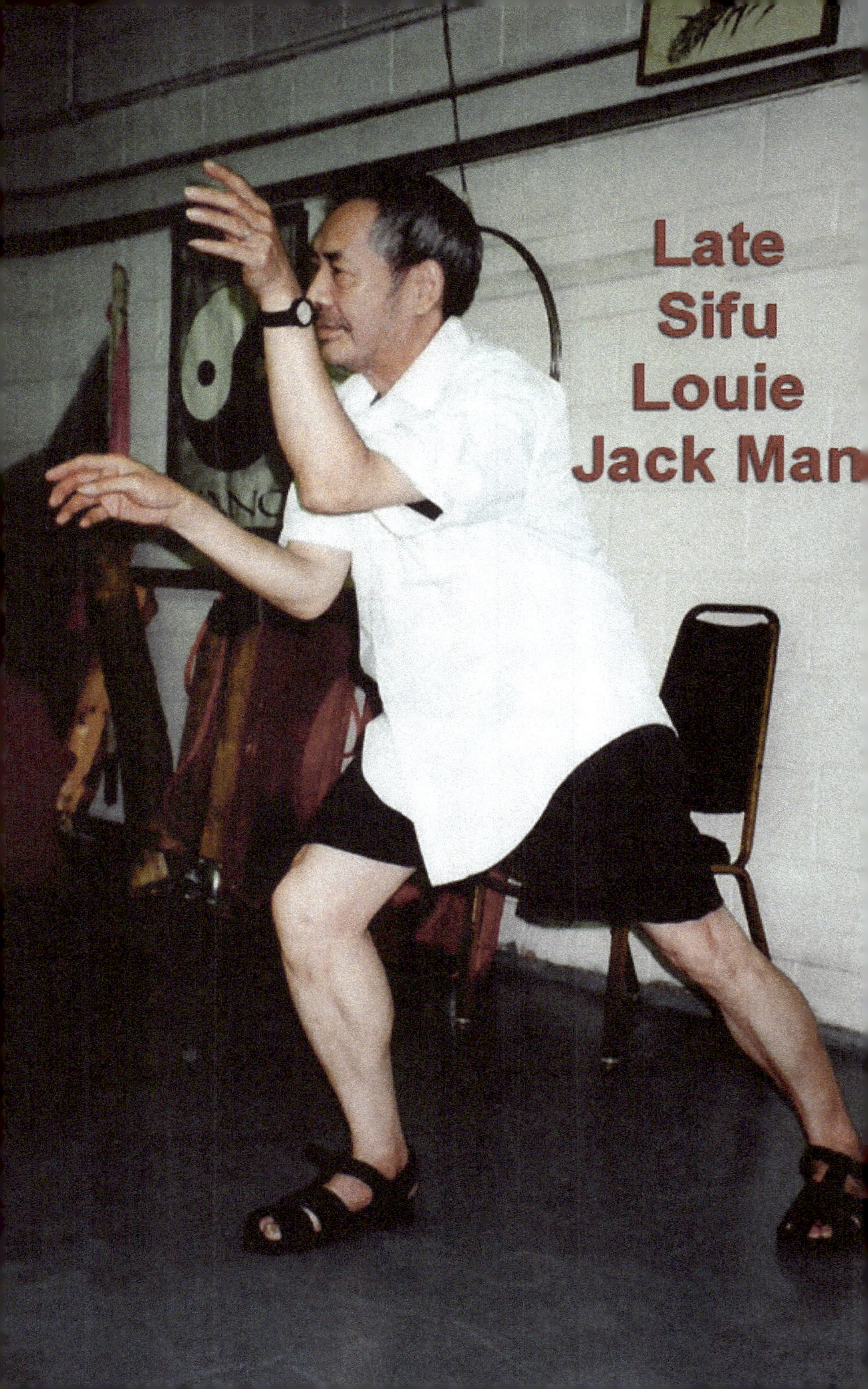

Late
Sifu
Louie
Jack Man

FEELING HAND NOT BUFFALO STRENGTH

Crossing hands one attempts to diffuse incoming forces by feeling and redirecting them. One should use refined force and technique and not rely on buffalo strength or brute force.

There is only one "ging-spring force" but expressed in 18 Buddha Hands:
Mor Ging, Gwak Ging, Choc Ging, etc

From the feet, waist and shoulders
power will arrive in the hands.

4 Word Secret of Ging Spring Power
Float - Ping Shu
Sink - Bao Zhang
Swallow - Gop Shu
Spit - Jet Shu

In essence, the 9 Defensive hands are Swallow and the 9 Offensive are spit. Float and Sink are functions of posture and ging.

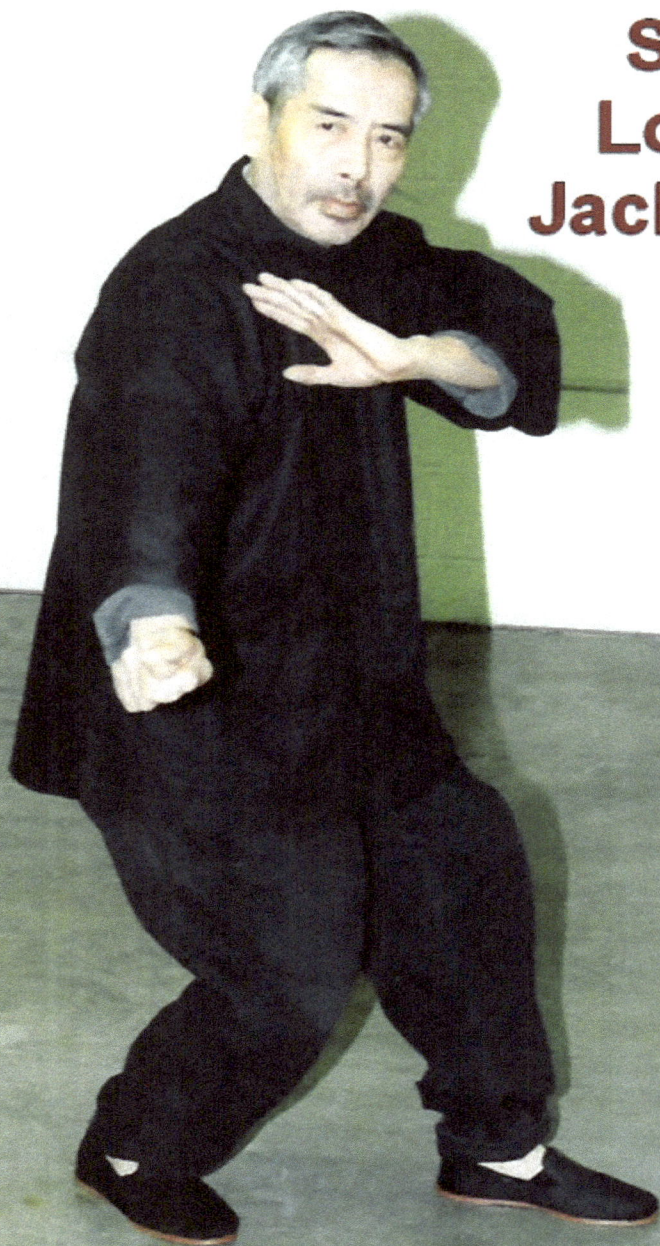
Late
Sifu
Louie
Jack Man

GING - SPRING POWER

Ging (Jing) is based on the Lik (natural strength) of a person but it is not natural. It is a refined strength, a strength that is acquired after special training. Martial art often speaks of "fa jing or fat ging", that is the issuing, emitting or sending forth of refined strength by various skills.

LIK AND GING POWER

Think of the body builder. He has both lik and ging. His natural strength (lik) is due to his body size and his refined strength (ging) is developed in the movement of lifting weights. Therefore, his ging is useful in moving weights. The person who digs ditches with a shovel will develop a refined power (ging) that allows him the greatest ease and comfort at shovelling. Use your (Lik) natural strength to refine kungfu explosive power (ging).

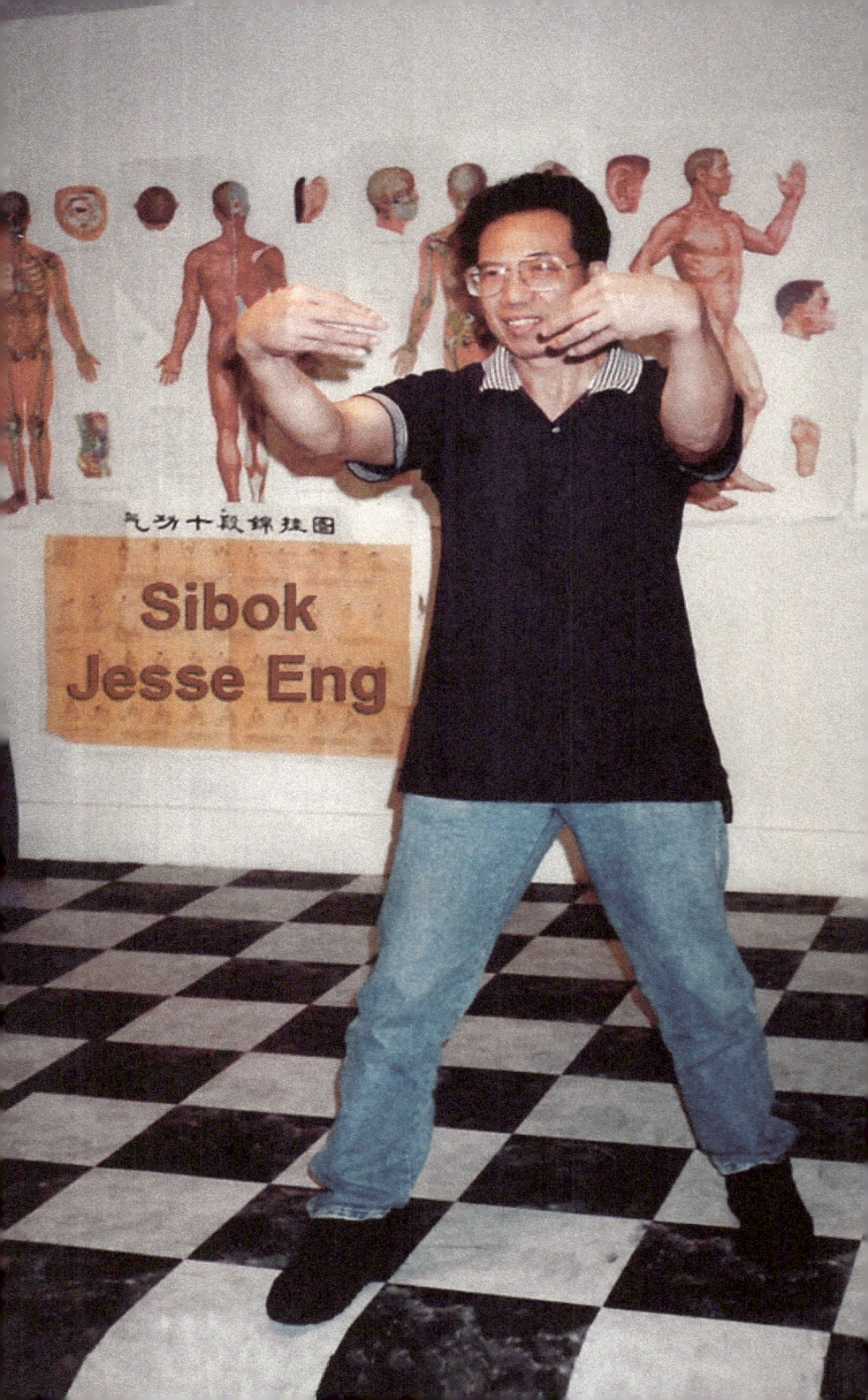

Sibok
Jesse Eng

气功十段锦庄图

DEAD GING POWER

If one's ging cannot be easily changed according to the opponent's reaction power and intent, then it is called "dead power". We see this in many Karate movements where force is met with greater force. It is "dead ging" because once exerted it usually cannot change or re-issue power until it has been regenerated usually by chambering or pulling back the hand as in the reverse punch.

LIVE GING POWER

In contrast, "live power or ging" strikes, sticks to, follows and regenerates power by using the opponents movement. The power is continuous and flowing without the need for pulling back the hand or recoiling the arm. One blow changes to another blow without ever breaking contact and always following the opponent's movement. This is refined in Hakka Mantis two man training.

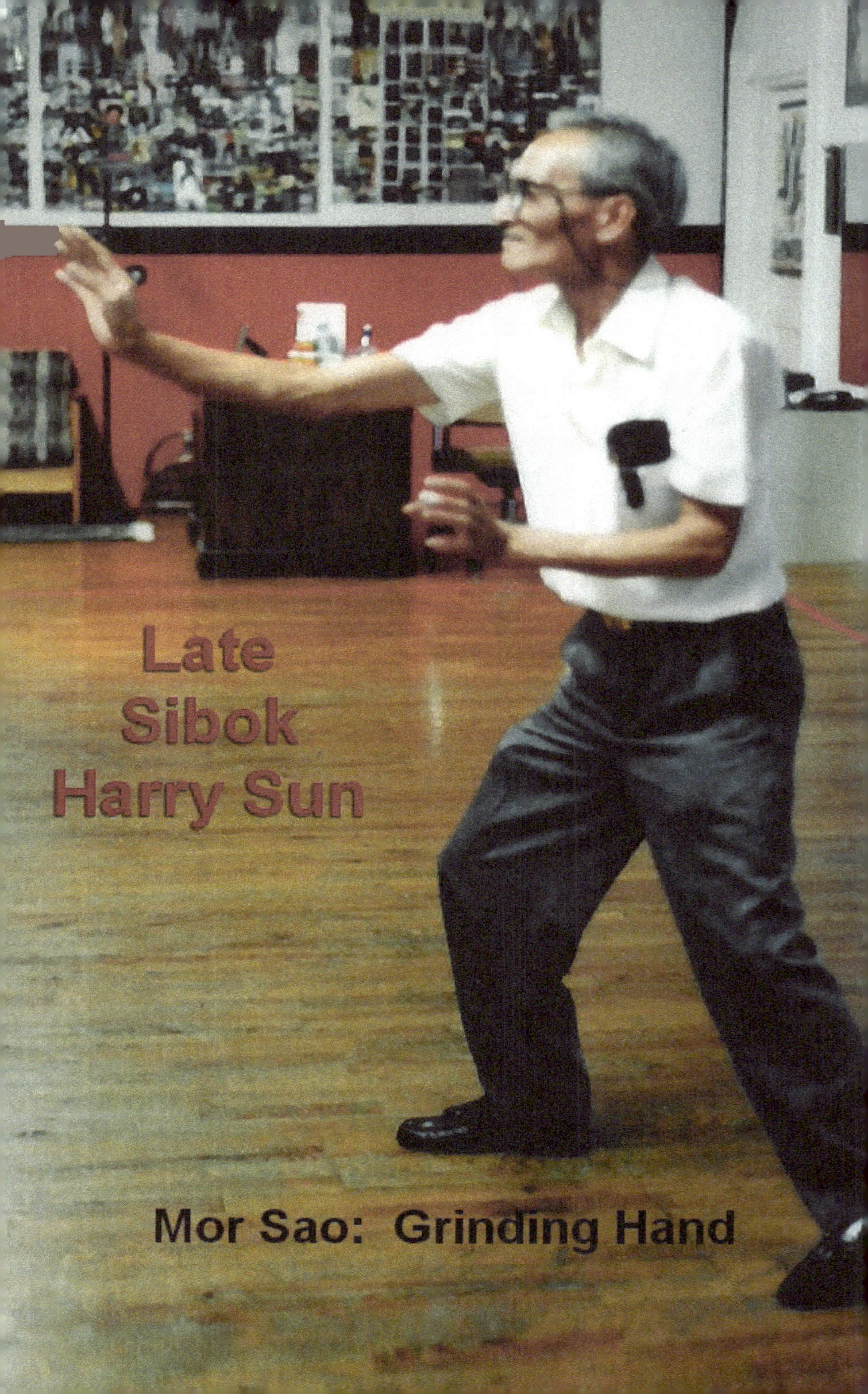

Late
Sibok
Harry Sun

Mor Sao: Grinding Hand

FOOTWORK

Correct horse is the father of power.
Mor Sao Grinding Hand is the mother of
hands.
Power is gathered through the feet and up
the legs and back, and expressed in the
hands. Without a firm stance there is no root
and without a root there will be little
power in the hands.

UP AND DOWN / FORWARD AND BACK

If the opponent is tall, I seem taller. If the
opponent is small, I seem smaller. Advancing to me he finds the distance long.
Retreating he finds the distance
exasperatingly short.

KEEP AND RETURN

Keep what comes in. Return what is going
away. Move in, make contact when there
is none. Give back what you get. With
one ounce one may return one thousand
pounds. Two tigers go separate ways
knowing both will be injured and
one may die.

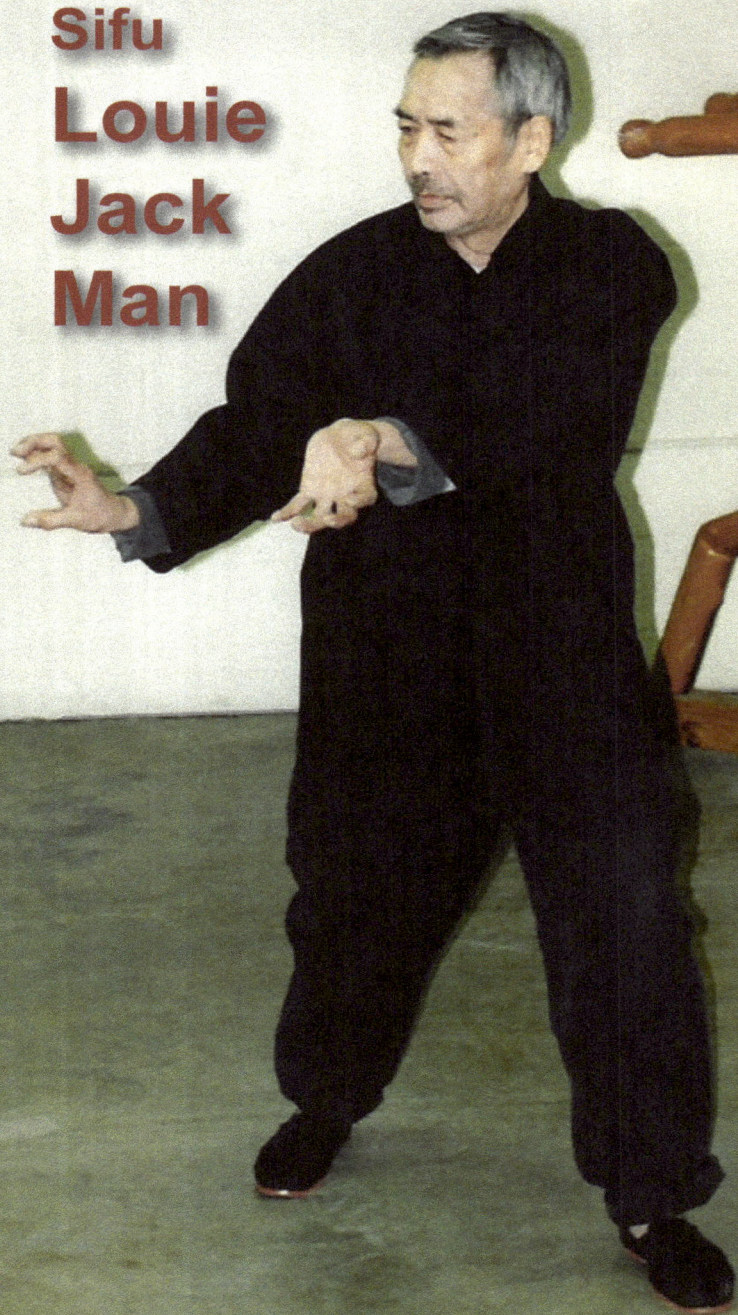

Late
Sifu
Louie
Jack
Man

HANDS ARE A PAIR OF DOORS

Open the doors you expose the center-line, close the doors and you protect it. Above the solar plexus is the upper gate, between it and the groin is the middle gate and below the groin is the lower gate. Opening and closing the centerline, you use hands I use hands, you use feet, I use feet.

SHOWING YOURSELF

When you show your temper, hold your hands. When you show your hand, hold your temper.

FISTS TO FACE

Visible fists strike invisible blows.

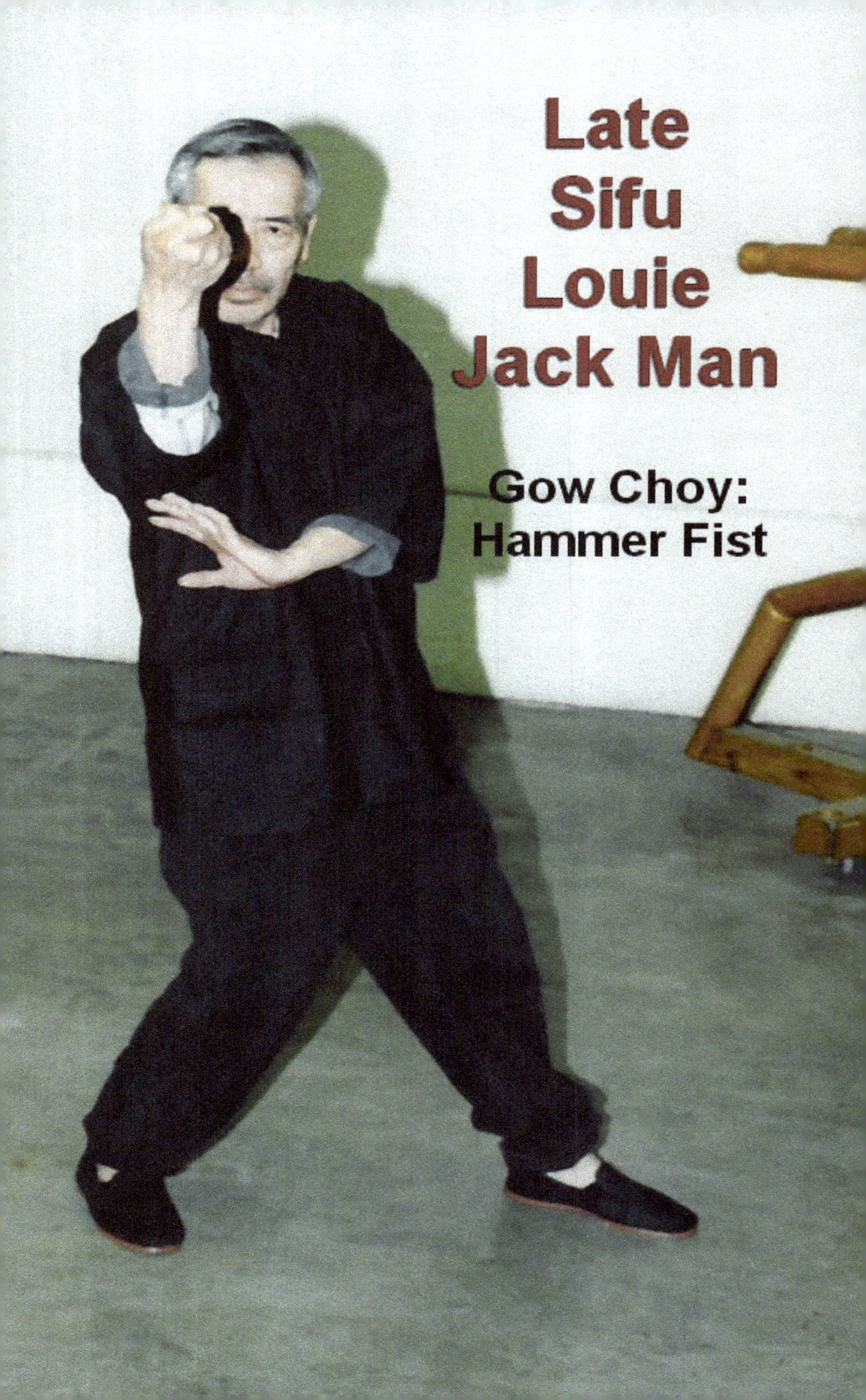

Late Sifu Louie Jack Man

Gow Choy: Hammer Fist

ONE ARM - THREE HANDS

Defend and attack with one arm is done by using the forearm for defensive movement while simultaneously attacking with the hand or fingers. This can only be accomplished if one has understood the centerline theory.

The mantis arm is composed of three "hands;" from the shoulder to the elbow, from the elbow to the wrist and from the wrist to the fingertips. A good mantis will use his "second hand" for control by pressing the forearm into the centerline of his prey, at the same time striking a vital area with his "first" hand or fingers.

ONE CONTROLS TWO
A skillful mantis will defend and attack using one arm to trap and control the opponents two arms, leaving one hand to attack freely at will.

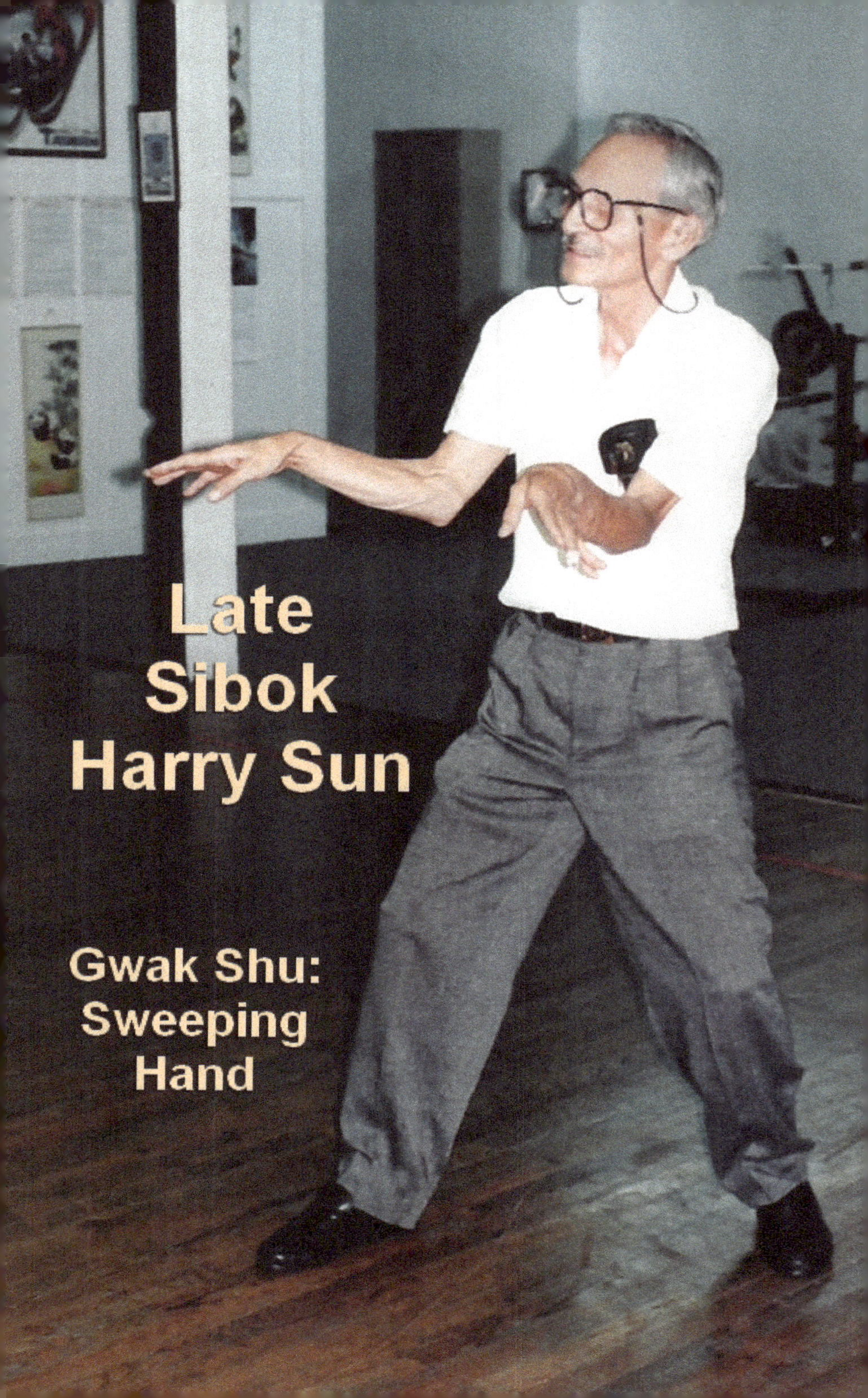

Late
Sibok
Harry Sun

Gwak Shu:
Sweeping
Hand

CONTACT, CONTROL, STRIKE

This principle of contact, control, and strike (until the opponent is red) is central to all Mantis action and is based on the three powers of the arm;
from the shoulder to the elbow, elbow to the wrist, wrist to the fingertips.

Contact - make a bridge
Control - borrow the opponent's force
Strike at will continuously

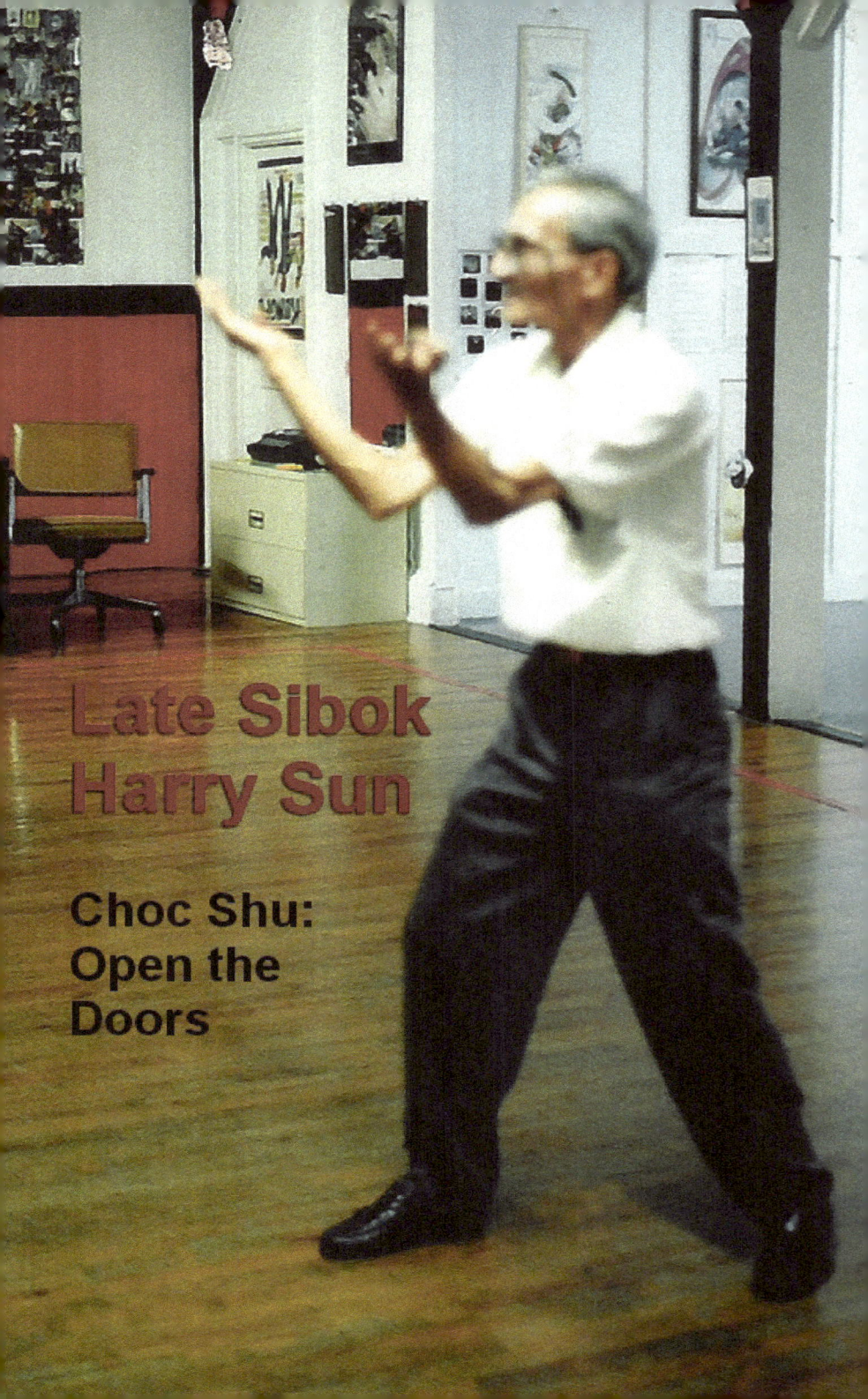

Late Sibok
Harry Sun

Choc Shu:
Open the
Doors

MANTIS TACTICS

A single movement of the arm
may contain several actions.

Tactical operations of the hand
include grappling, catching, holding,
capturing, clasping with the forearms,
slicing strikes with the knuckles, pressing
with the elbow, sudden quick pushes with
both hands, spearing with extended fingers, flicking of the hands in quick jabs,
exploding fingers from the fists, jerking
the opponent's arm, slicing and chopping
with the edge of the palm, hooking and
deflecting hands, elbow strikes, claw-like
raking actions, and poking with the back
of the hands. Many of the movements
are simultaneously
defensive and offensive.

The feet, ankles, knees and hips may
mirror the hand movements.

Late
Sibok
Harry Sun

Sai Shu:
Roller Arm

STICKY HAND

Sticky training is to learn relaxation.

It is the ability to not blink when being struck.

It is attaching to the center
of the opponent's being, neither pushing
into nor pulling away from him.

It is being perfectly attacthed in
stillness and motion.

Feeling hand is the result of sticky hand.

One must learn to neither anticipate the
opponent's movement or
telegraph his own.

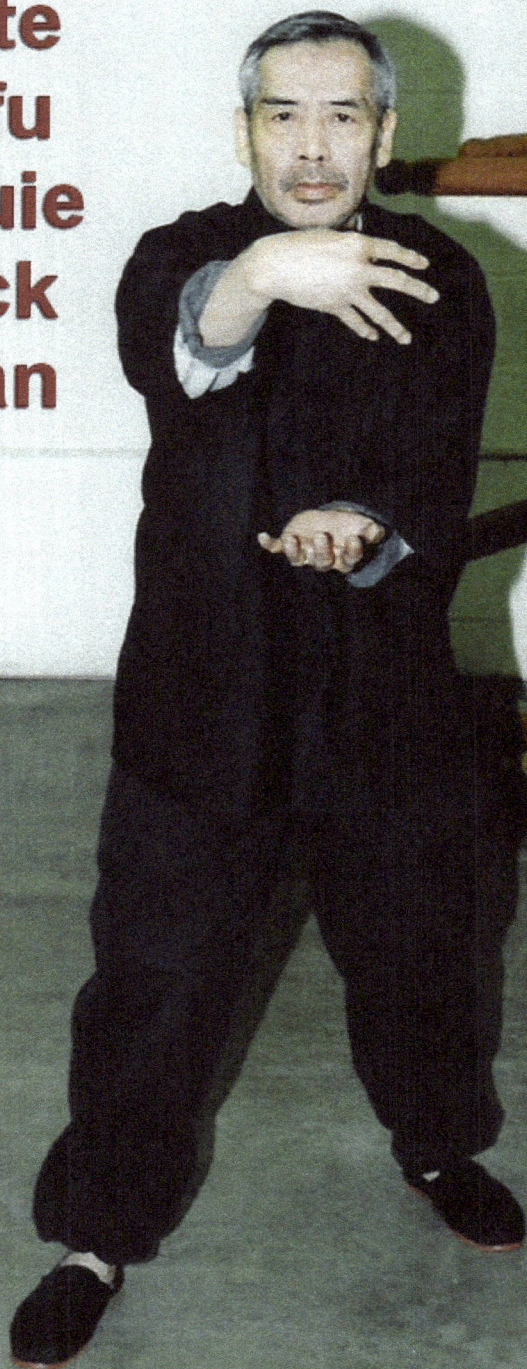

Late
Sifu
Louie
Jack
Man

Han Shu:
Slice
Deflect
Attack

FEELING HAND

Feeling hand is the reading
of the opponents intent. It is as if the
hand (body) has an eye of its own.

Controlling hand is the result of feeling
hand. It is the jamming, trapping and
deflecting and attacking of the opponents
intent. This is done based on the control
points of the body.

The motto, is
"hand to hand, heart to heart,
you don't come, I won't start."

(The hands are placed (chambered)
above the heart and the elbows cover the
ribcage to protect the internal organs).

Two man training is to know others.
Single man shadowboxing is to
know one's self.

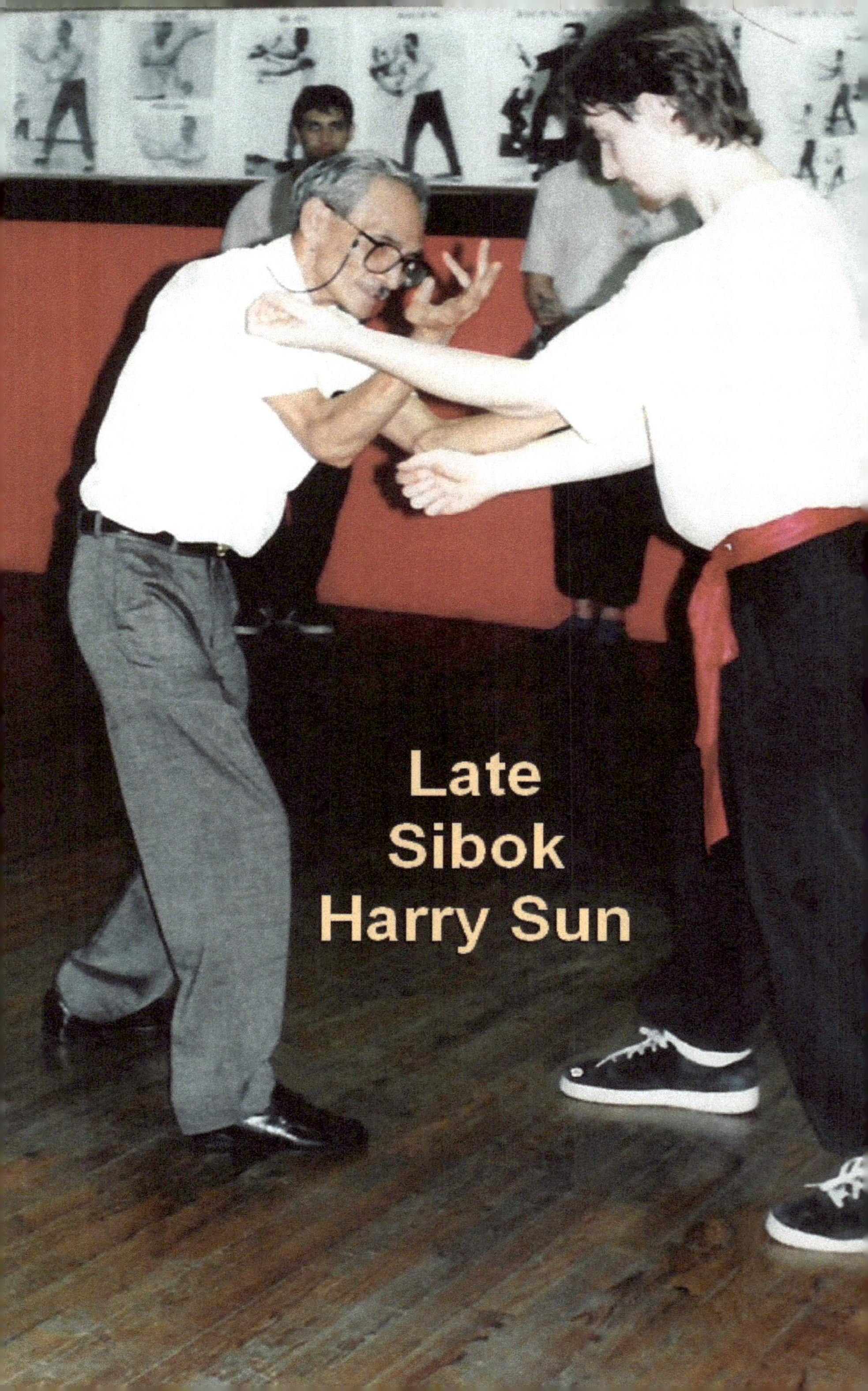

Late
Sibok
Harry Sun

BRIDGING, RANGE, DISTANCE

A bridge is any part of the body used to close the distance to the opponent. Arm and hands are commonly the bridge. Single, Double, Triple bridging is possible using hands and feet.

Three methods are hard bridge (smash through the opponent); soft bridge (borrowing force); and evasive bridge in which contact with the opponent is avoided or neutralized. Any and each of the 18 offensive and defensive hands may be used as a bridge and their turning power then used for immediate striking.

If there exists a bridge then cross the bridge. If no bridge exists then make a bridge. If under the bridge then return to the top. If on top of the bridge stay on top and immediately cross. Regular training may make one aggressive in nature. The constant rubbing, feeling, and turning of power acquired during feeding hands gives one confidence to defeat the enemy.

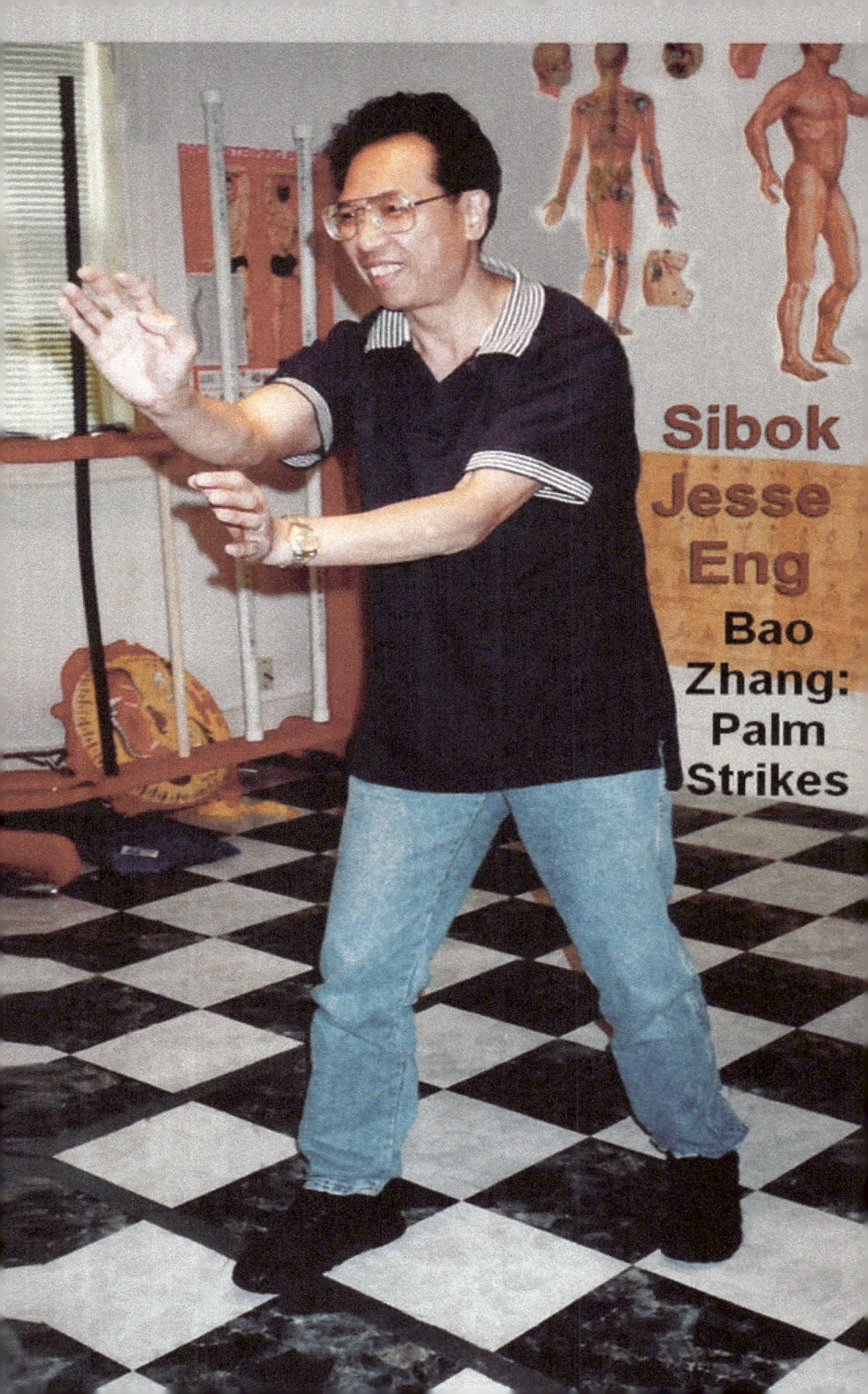

Sibok Jesse Eng

Bao Zhang: Palm Strikes

SOLO TRAINING

Although, Hakka mantis combat is only mastered by two man (paired training) the essential skills must be thoroughly trained and made ones own through solo training.

One must individually set a personal schedule and exercise himself daily until the fundamental skills, basics, single man forms, apparatus, and weapons are instinctually understood.

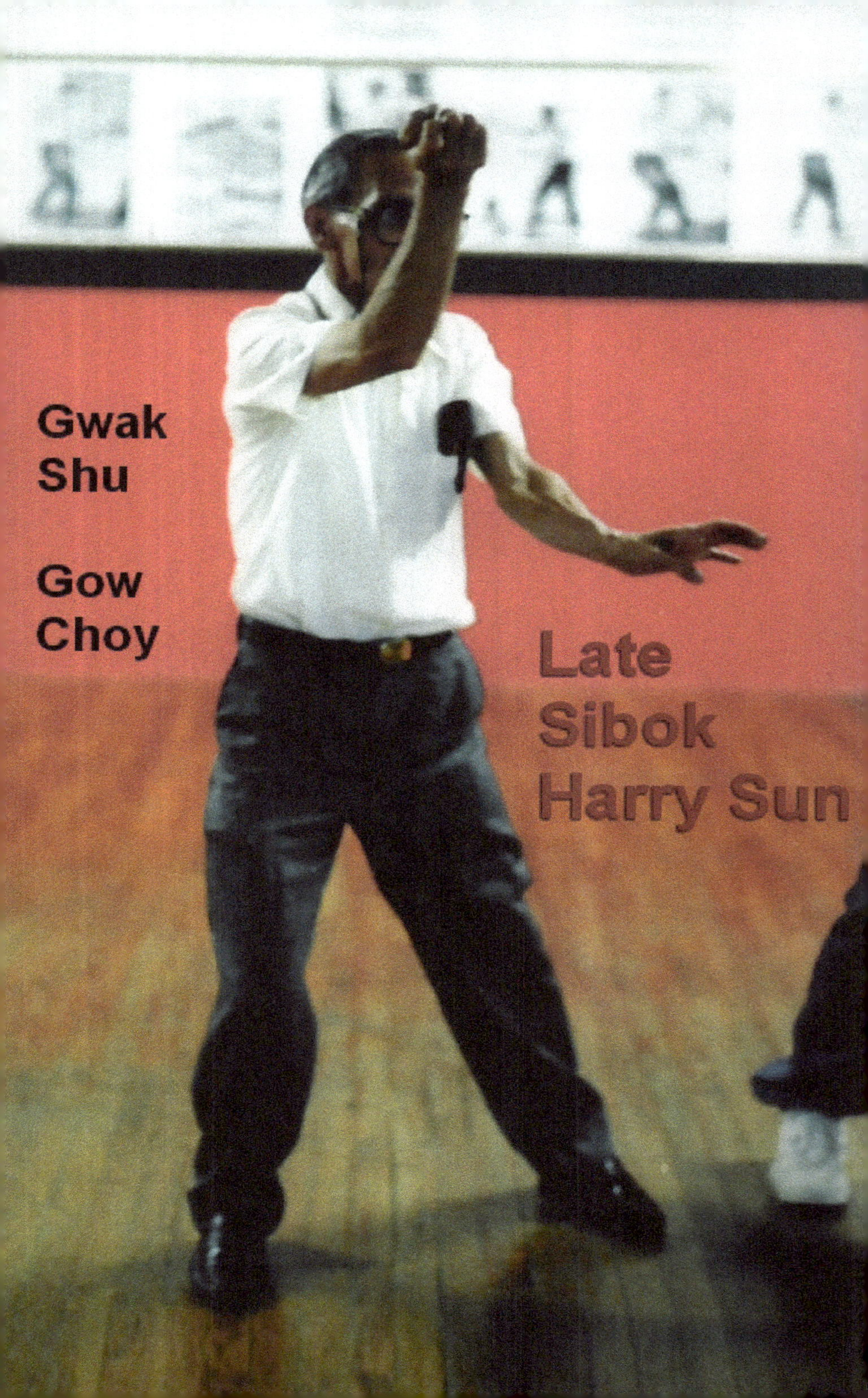

Gwak
Shu

Gow
Choy

Late
Sibok
Harry Sun

PAIRED TRAINING

Self Defense requires two man training to be realistic and cannot be learned by shadowboxing alone.

Paired training methods are numerous from basic conditioning, strengthening, one - three - nine steps, sticky hands, sticky legs, sticky body, to the advanced two man sets and vital point target practice.

Don't hang your meat on their hook, is the Hakka saying. This means borrow the opponent's force but do not give him yours.

Give yourself up to follow others and your hand will accurately weigh their force and your feet will measure the distance of their approach without mistake.

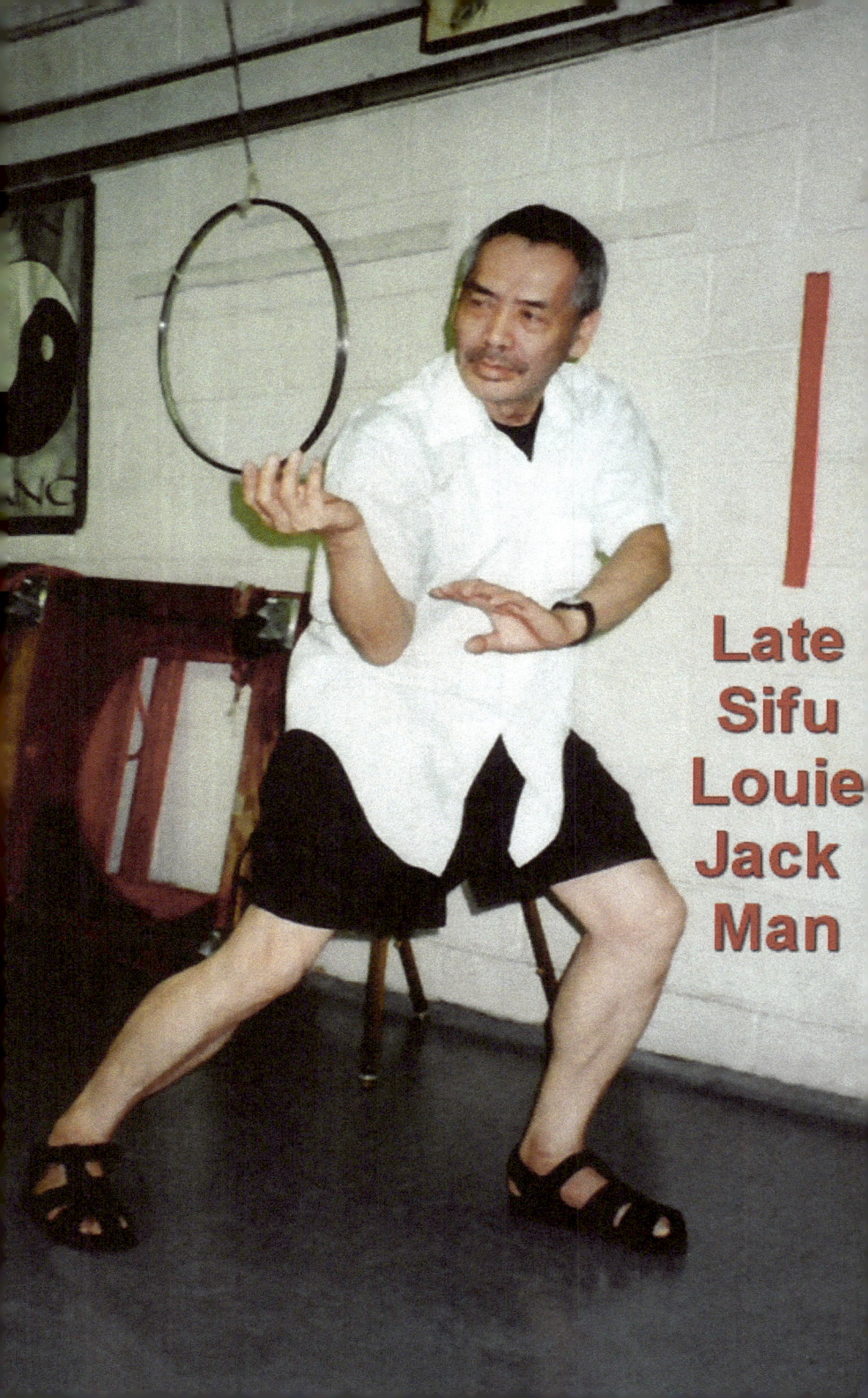

Late
Sifu
Louie
Jack
Man

VITAL POINT TRAINING

Variations in locating the points exist. Using the distance of one's finger width, each spot may be located.

Some say from the head to the toe about every one inch contains a large spot and every 10th of an inch a small spot.

Chinese kungfu usually at the deepest level, speaks of these 36 large spots and 72 small spots —108.

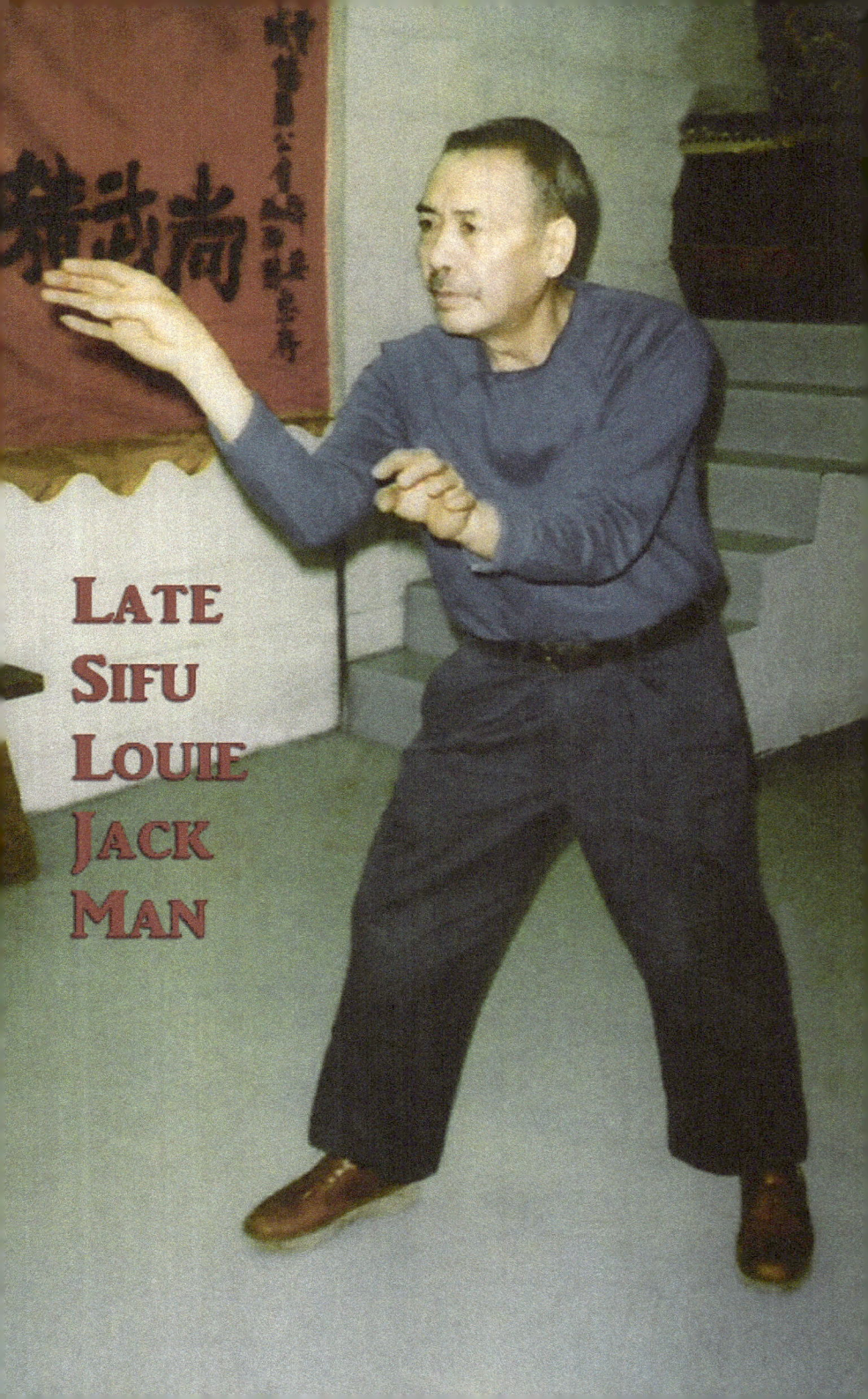

LATE
SIFU
LOUIE
JACK
MAN

HAKKA MARTIAL MAXIM

When drinking water, one should drink
as close to the source as possible, as
the water becomes murky and often
polluted the further down stream
one travels.

I encourage you to seek out the plain
truth for yourself.

Do not follow anyone blindly.

Search and prove all things!

Doubt everything.
Find your own light. - S. Gautama

Abridged Southern Mantis History in China

CHINA HAKKA MANTIS HISTORY

Monk Som Dot's two disciples transmit
three Orders of Shaolin Praying Mantis Kungfu

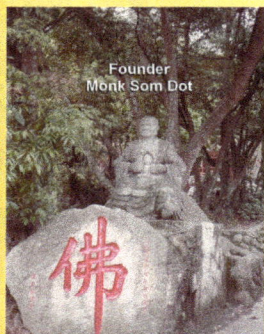

Founder
Monk Som Dot

It is said that Monk Som Dot was originally from Tibet and that he wandered extensively studying Shaolin boxing and medicine.

At the invitation of the Taoist Pope he travelled to Kwongsai Mt. Dragon Tiger and after settling there, he accepted two disciples, Wong Leng, an illiterate, but diligent disciple, and Lee Siem. Lee Siem later became known as Siem Yuen, which means capable of grasping the depth of Buddhism. And Wong Leng became known as Wong Do Yuen, capable in Taoism.

After some years, Som Dot sent his two disciples down the mountain to spread his art of Shaolin, which was divided into three orders. The first order taught the principle of 10 soft and one hard, and was taught only on the top of the mountain. The second order was half hard, half soft power. The third order was based on extremely forceful techniques. This is the reason the art is sometimes called a "three door or gate" art today.

In doing so, as they descended the mountain, Wong Do Yuen and Lee Siem Yuen, at the middle gate of the mountain, accepted a student named Chu Long Bot. Hiding the kungfu of the first order, they taught Chu Long Bot only the second order kungfu of Som Dot. At that time, the first order kungfu of Som Dot was not taught.

After learning the art, Chu, having no knowledge of the first order kungfu, betrayed Wong and Lee and used only the Chu surname to pass on what became 'Chu Gar Gao' - Chu Family Creed. The name was later changed again to "Chu Gar Praying

Mantis" in Hong Kong.

Chu Long Bot later taught Chu An Nam, who taught Yang Sao and Lao Sui, who was a friend of Chu Kwei, who was the father of Chu Kwong Hua in contemporary times. This order of kungfu was originally taught only at the middle gate of the mountain.

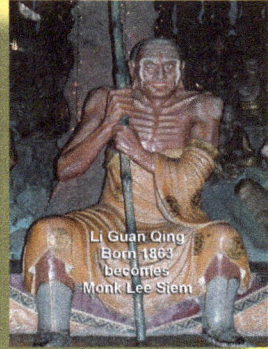

Li Guan Qing Born 1863 becomes Monk Lee Siem

Later, as Wong Do Yuen and Lee Siem Yuen went back down the mountain, at the lower gate, a praying mantis insect popped out in front of them. Wong, being the first to step off the mountain, proclaimed the mantis must be a sign from Heaven and to avoid further persecution of Som Dot's Shaolin teaching, the Shaolin art of three orders should simply be called Praying Mantis.

At the bottom of the mountain, a man surnamed Choy and nicknamed Tit Ngau, or Iron Ox, pleaded with sincerity to learn their kungfu and the two of them taught him Som Dot's third order of kungfu based on extremely forceful techniques.

Not knowing what to call the art, Choy, having no knowledge of the first or second order of Som Dot, eventually did the same as the Chu Clan and called the art Tit Ngau, or Iron Ox. Later a fellow named Chung Lo Ku learned from Choy and passed on this teaching as Chung Gar Gao in the East River region. This kungfu of the third order was taught at the bottom of the mountain.

In China, it is said each of Som Dot's three orders of Shaolin Kungfu has its advantage and each is worthwhile to learn and study.

Author's note: For an in-depth look at the origins and history of Southern Praying Mantis in China refer to the book, *Pingshan Mantis Celebration,* from SouthernMantisPress.com. Also, refer to the five volume eBook, *China Southern Praying Mantis Kung Survey*™ at chinamantis.com. (Monk Images are representations only; Som Dot left and Lee Siem above.)

Note on Hand Names and Translations

In China, everyone has their own "jia xiang hua", or village dialect. Hakka is one such dialect and each clan or town may even have their own pronunciation of Hakka language. The names given herein are the names that are commonly used so that everyone is on the same page and understands which skill or hand is being talked about. It is less important what you call the skills, and more important that everyone understands. The Chinese romanization herein is the same—it is written phonetically or what is common, so that it can be easily understood. Chinese names herein are not correct pinyin, purposely.

"Shu, Sao, and Shou" all simply mean "hand" and are often used interchangeably. Remember, once the stance, root and feeling hand is skilled, the whole body is one "hand".

About Southern Mantis on the Internet

The internet and DVDs can be a great aid to learning. How much better are DVDs than secretly peeking through holes in a fence or wall to learn Mantis? In the early days, sneaking a peek through a hole was quite common.

Nothing can replace the spirit and hand of a skillful teacher. But, the new media and resources are still a valuable asset. The internet, however, is also a large source of disinformation. Repeating what someone else said erroneously often becomes accepted as SPM "truth" without verification. There is a great deal of "false" information on the internet about Southern Praying Mantis.

An example is the 'Blanco' article. Circa mid 1990s, Blanco, from Hong Kong, called my office in the USA asking how to contact Southern Mantis teachers in China. I did not provide him any information. Southern Mantis teachers usually frown on unannounced visits from strangers. Later, he "compiled" his article using sources, such as my published works, without permission. Much of his article is erroneous and needs correction. I encourage you to seek the truth for yourself. Do not follow any one blindly. Search and prove all things. The further you go downstream the murkier the water. Drink close to the source.

About the Photographs in this Book
The images are from my personal library. They were not made in a studio for glamor, but made on the spot with the various Teachers herein. Appreciate the images for what they are - natural shots of Sifu, in their own elements. None of the images can be made again—those days are gone. Sadly, many of the elder teachers have passed away, as well.

A Final Note

If you are interested in Southern Praying Mantis boxing, then I encourage you to read all of my books. They are genuine books of the true heritage of Southern Mantis. And although they are written by me, I can't really call them mine. I am just a transmitter of the heritage.

The branches of Southern Praying Mantis are from one root. Each has its advantage and is worthy of study. Although, I am first, Kwongsai Jook Lum Temple Mantis, and second, Chu Gar Mantis, both by Ceremony and Transmission, I am not biased or preferential. They are harmonious and may be taught side by side. The only difference is the depth of the transmission one receives.

Email me if you have a question, suggestion, or specific topic of Southern Praying Mantis you'd like addressed.

If you are interested in training by DVD or coming to Hong Kong - China to study Southern Mantis, then you may email me directly. I have a class in Guangdong, China, Cheng Chiu Sifu, teaches Chu Gar and Hakka Unicorn culture in Hong Kong and Wong Yu Hua Sifu's Guang Wu Tang is open. Welcome!

Roger D. Hagood
Standing Chairman
Bamboo Temple Chinese Benevolent Association, USA
Hong Kong Chu Gar Tonglong Martial Art Association
rdh@chinamantis.com

Vol 1: Pingshan Mantis Celebration Hardcover or eBook

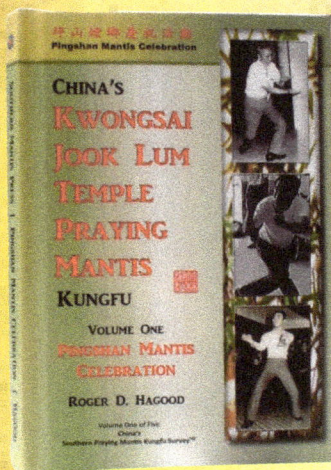

Pingshan Mantis Celebration
A rare book of China's Kwongsai Jook Lum Temple Praying Mantis Kungfu and Unicorn Culture.

Included are: Origins, history and practices of China's Kwongsai Mantis, rare and exclusive historical photographs never published before, the hometown of Kwongsai Mantis-Pingshan Town, how Wong Yuk Kong came to learn Hakka Mantis, why Wong Sifu went "mad" after a spell was cast, why Hakka Mantis is divided into "three orders" and what they are, three Wong Brothers who inherited Kwongsai Mantis, what Kwongsai Mantis boxing was taught early on and now, what happened when Kwongsai Mantis and Chu Gar first met, Hakka Mantis descending the mountain on horseback in 1917, English and Chinese translation of how Master Chung blossomed Hakka Mantis in South China, Hakka Culture along the East River, extensive interviews with inheritor Wong

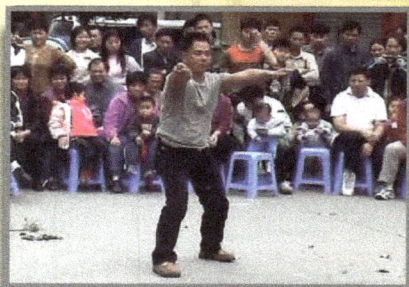

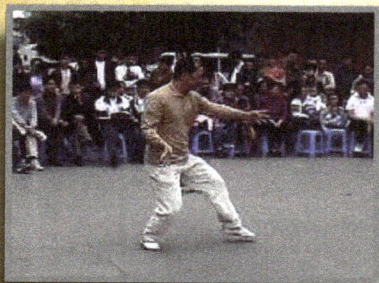

Yu Hua about sensitive topics, rules and regulations of Wong Yuk Kong's Mantis School, a Hakka Feast in Pingshan Town, valuable Hakka Mantis resources online and off, Hakka Mantis boxing maxims and proverbs, dozens of Kwongsai Mantis boxing postures, staff, and sword pictures, rare never before published Jook Lum Mantis reliquary photographs, the Bamboo Forest Temple true heritage Dit Da liniment prescription and more.

116

Hardcover Collector's Edition Book

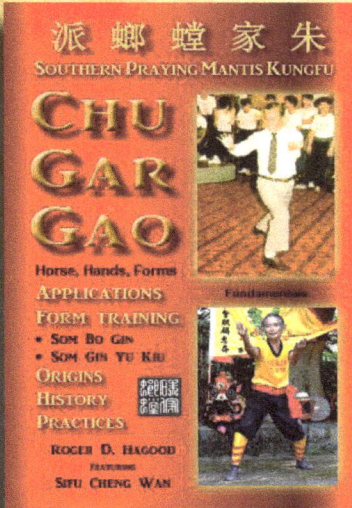

Chu Gar Gao: Southern Mantis
A rare treatise of Hakka Chu Gar Southern Praying Mantis boxing that includes: Chu Gar Mantis history, boxing transmission, six Chu Gar areas, three kinds of Chu Gar in China; Chu Gar Mantis personal records --- Sifu Chen Ching Hong, Sifu Yip Sui, Sifu Cheng Wan, Sifu Cheng Chiu, Sifu Dong Yat Long, Sifu Ma Jiuhua, Past Masters in Charge; Chu Gar applications --- Single Bridge Tsai Sao, Double Bridge Dui Jong, Mang Dan Sao Dui Jong, Ying Sao Shadow Hand, Gow Choy Hammer Fist, Locking Hands, Bridge, Tan Sao, and Ginger Fist, Double Bridge Gwak Sao, Sticky Hand and Intercepting Hand Bao Zhang Palms; Chu Gar shadowboxing forms in pictorial--Som Bo Gin (Three Step Arrow) and Som Gin Yu Kiu (Three Arrows Shaking Bridge form); and more.

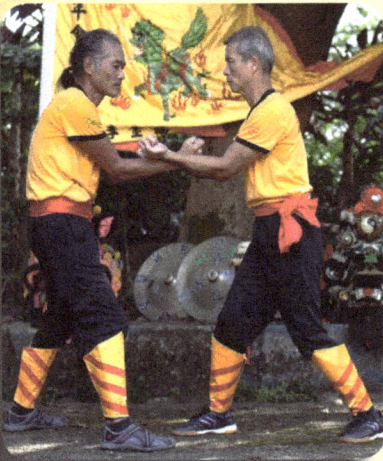

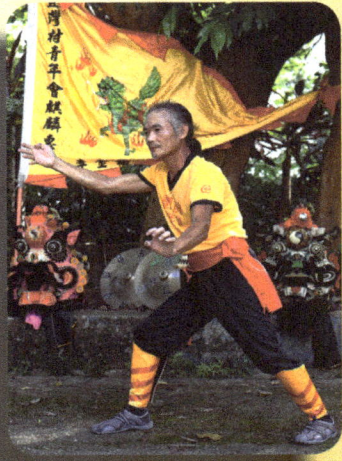

Available at Amazon, Barnes and Noble, and other fine booksellers!
Search Keywords - Southern Mantis Press

VOL 2, 3, 4: China Mantis Survey Hardcover or eBook

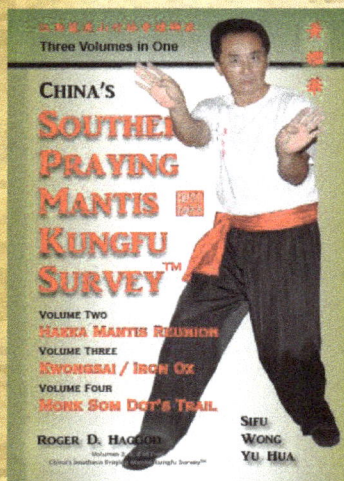

A rare three volume book of China's Hakka Kwongsai Jook Lum Temple and Iron Ox Praying Mantis boxing.

Volume Two, China Hakka Mantis Reunion, includes: Three Orders of Som Dot's Shaolin Mantis revisited, Hakka Mantis blossoms in Huizhou, Elder Lok Wei Ping-a Chu Gar and Kwongsai Sifu, Chung Yel Chong teaches one form, Kwongsai and Chu Gar clash in the 40s, Sifu Wong Gok Hong takes the lion head away, Lau Say Kay Sifu plays non-standard Kwongsai Mantis, Sifu Lai Wei Keung first Instructor in 1948, One Kwongsai form originally taught, Two methods of beggar hands, Sifu Cho Gum, Sifu Wong Yu Hua, Fairy hands cause a slap on the rear, Lok Sifu plays 34 Plum Blossom Staff, All Mantis is one family, Lai Sifu plays 34 Plum Blossom staff and more!

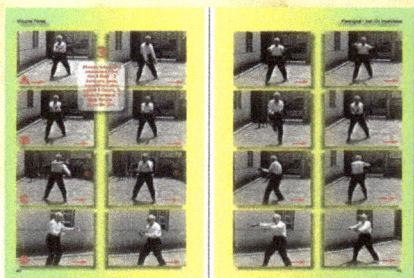

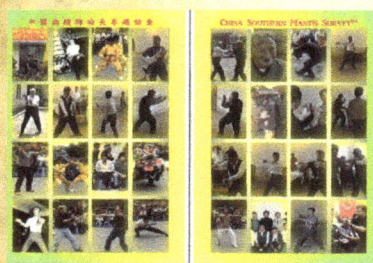

Volume Three, Kwongsai / Iron Ox Interviews, includes: Records of the elders and knowledge lost, Sifu Yao Kam Fat, Wong Yuk Kong opens Kwongsai Mantis in Hong Kong, Wong Yuk Kong visits Lao Sui's Chu Gar school, Wong Yuk Kong defeats 10 assailants, Yao Sifu plays three steps-three scisscors old form, Similarities in Hakka Mantis, Yao Sifu plays 34 Plum Blossom staff, Spirit Shrine of Wong Yuk Kong, Elder Sifu Chung Wu Xing first disciple

VOL 2, 3, 4: Three Volumes in One Hardcover Book

of Chung Yel Chong, Iron Uncle Chung friend of Lam Sang, Iron Uncle Chung smokes opium with Lam Sang and Master Chung in the 1930s, Sifu Yang Gun Ming student of Chung Yel Chong, Dit Da Doctors by lineage, Hakka Mantis prohibited in the Cultural Revolution, Sifu Xu Men Fei Iron Ox Hakka Mantis, Iron Ox taught only 2 months a year, Xu Sifu plays Iron Ox Second Door form-Red Flag Staff-and Third Door form, Iron Ox challenges Wong Yuk Kong's Kwongsai Mantis, Iron Ox Secret Drill Hand not taught, and more.

Note: The hardcover book has supplemental information not contained in the eBook.

Volume Four, On Monk Som Dot's Trail / Chung Yel Chong Family Interviews, includes: Sifu Chung Wei Fei grandson of Master Chung, Master Chung Yel Chong as a boy accepted by Monk Lee, Chung Go Wah son of third ancestor Master Chung, Master Chung's boxing and Dit Da Medicine books, Third Ancestor Chung teaches Kwongsai Mantis in Hong Kong 1920s, Master Chung kills a man in self-defense, Master Chung's three generations under one roof, Sifu Lee Kok Leung outlines his Kwongsai Mantis teaching, Sifu Patrick Lee plays Mantis in Pingshan Town, Lee Sifu's History of Kwongsai Mantis, On Som Dot's Trail - Shanxi Jook Lum Temple, Oldest of the Temple Halls, Chung and Monk Lee return South six months on horseback, Kwongsai Dragon Tiger Mountain of Shaolin boxing and spiritualism, The bottom line about Kwongsai Jook Lum Temple, Lam Sang's Kwongsai spiritualism and amulet, Monk Lee Siem looks like a ghost, Jook Lum Temple in Hong Kong, Jook Lum Temple in Macau, Map of Jook Lum Temples in China with Hakka Mantis boxing, Abridged China Hakka Mantis history, Guang Wu Tang Martial Hall of Wong Yuk Kong in 2012, Mission statement of Guang Wu Tang Kwongsai Mantis, Sifu Wong Yu Hua in 2012, Miscellanies, Resources, Train in China. Kwongsai Mantis and Iron Ox boxing and staff forms in sequence, and more.

- Hardcover
- Full color
- 330+ photographs
- 128 pages

Available at Amazon, Barnes and Noble, and other fine booksellers!
Search Keywords - Southern Mantis Press

Hardcover Collector's Edition Book

Eighteen Buddha Hands
Kwongsai Jook Lum Temple Mantis

A rare instructional treatise of Chinese boxing from the Kwongsai Dragon-Tiger Mountain, Bamboo Forest Temple, Praying Mantis Clan, as transmitted by the late Grandmaster Lam Sang.

Details include stories of Lam Sang's supernatural ability such as Poison Snake Staff, Sun Gazing, and Light Body Skills. Boxing principles elaborated are Body posture, Rooting, Sinking, Center-line, Spiral power, Contact-control-strike, Intercepting and sticky hand, Bridging, Anticipating-telegraphing, Dead and live power, Form and function, 4 word secret, Dim Mak vital points and more.

Boxing Fundamentals included are Footwork: Chop, Circle, Advance, Shuffle step, Turnarounds, Side to side; Kicks, Sweeps, Takedowns, Grappling, Chin Na Seizing, Hook hands, Elbow strokes, Dui Jong, Sticky hands, Forms, and Phases of training. Eighteen Buddha Hand techniques, 9 defensive, 9 offensive, are illustrated in color with instruction in attributes, function and vital point targeting. Boxing maxims of strategy and tactics are included.

Available at Amazon, Barnes and Noble, and other fine booksellers!
Search Keywords - Southern Mantis Press

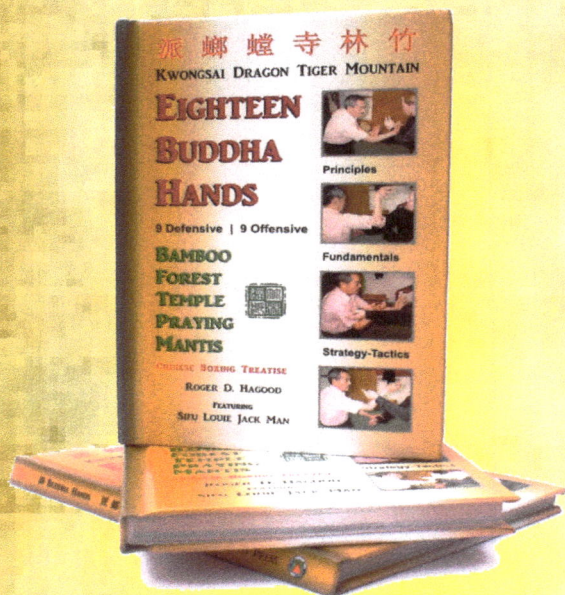

MantisFlix™ Video eBooks

60 Years of Southern Mantis Movies and Events!

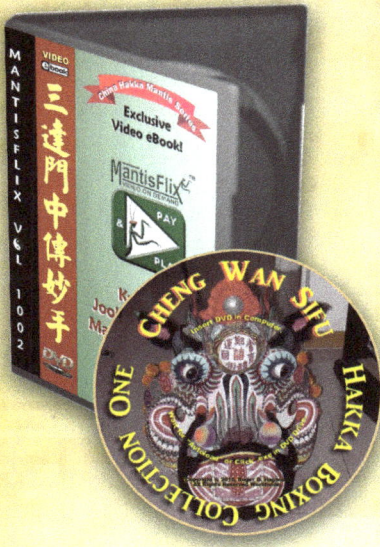

Wong Fei Hong and the Jook Lum Temple

Volume 1001 - Hong Kong 1954

B/W Classic Movie Exclusive! 100,000 plus clip previews on YouTube. Get your full copy now!

Kwongsai Mantis Celebration

Volume 1002 - Pingshan Town, Guangdong, China

Late Sifu Wong Yuk Kong Kwongsai Jook Lum Clan 35th Anniversary Celebration, circa 2003.

Hakka Boxing Collection One
Volume 1003 - A rare collection of Hakka Boxing.

Hakka Boxing Collection Two
Volume 1004 - A second rare collection of Hakka Boxing.

Chu Gar Cheng Wan Celebration
Volume 1005 - Join the 1989 Cheng Wan Chu Gar Mantis Celebration in Hong Kong! Cheng Wan Sifu was the inheritor of Chu Gar descended from Lao Sui.

View and Enjoy Video Previews Online:
www.MantisFlix.com

Our Family of Hakka Mantis Websites
Visit and Enjoy!
Informational, Educational, Instructive

A ten year ongoing research in China of the origins, history and practices of Southern Mantis!
Dedicated to the late Wong Yuk Kong Sifu in China!
chinamantis.com

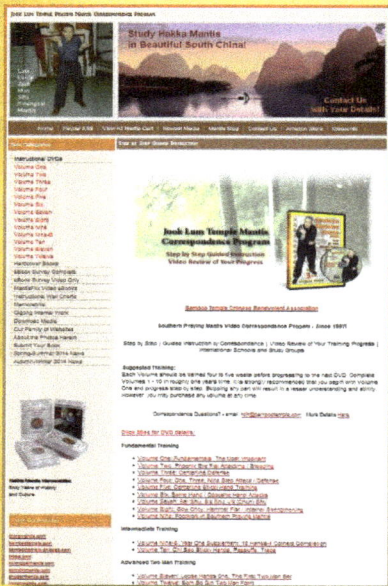

The Bamboo Temple Association is a mutual aid fraternity.Join us and become a member, School, Branch or Study Group today!Dedicated to the late Lam Sang Sifu's teaching in the USA.
bambootemple.com
btcba.com

These sites reveal many China Kwongsai Mantis Sifu who have heretofore remained silent about the teaching of Kwongsai Dragon Tiger Mountain Bamboo Forest Temple Mantis and outlay the lineage of Hakka Mantis as stated in China.
kwongsaimantis.com
somdotmantis.com

This site details the complete history of Chu Gar Gao Hakka Praying Mantis as descended from the late Lao Sui in Hong Kong and Hui Yang (Wai Yearn), China.

Resources

(con't) Dedicated to the late Cheng Wan Sifu who passed in 2009.
chugarmantis.com

This site is dedicated to the late Xu Fat Chun Sifu and speaks of the history of Iron Ox Hakka Praying Mantis in Pingdi Town, Guangdong, China.
ironoxmantis.com

Historical Hakka Mantis Flix! Some 60+ years of Hakka Southern Praying Mantis Kungfu movies and events in video eBooks!
mantisflix.com

Our dedicated South Mantis Tube. We have several hundreds of hours of videos in our Hakka Mantis archives dating back to 1950 in China that we hope to share with you!Feel free to share.Upload your Southern Mantis or Hakka video now!
southmantis.com

Genuine Internal Work - the original 11 month correspondence course of Tien Tao Qigong.
tientaoqigong.com

Ancient Methods to achieve vitality and a healthier well-being! The Oriental Secrets Series of Qigong.
oss.tientaoqigong.com

And our YouTube channel:
youtube.com/chinamantissurvey

Memorabilia from Southern Mantis Press.com

Southern Mantis Instructional Playing Cards

Kwongsai Mantis
18 Buddha Hands

Card Backs: Various Sifu of Lam Sang's generations in multiple postures

Card Fronts: Two man application photos, Text instruction, Instructive maxims

Includes the 18 Buddha Hands and more of Kwongsai Hakka Mantis

Key Benefits
of our Card Decks

- 54 Cards with Hakka Mantis
- Customized Front and Back
- Full Vibrant Color!
- Instructional
- Educational
- Informative
- Rare and Exclusive Content and Photographs
- Entertaining - Play Hakka Mantis Cards with your friends

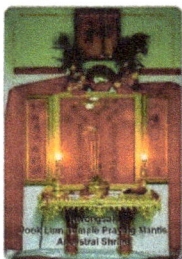
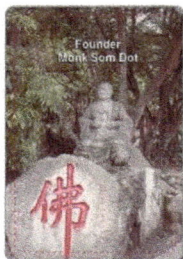
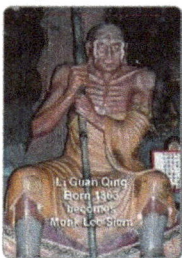
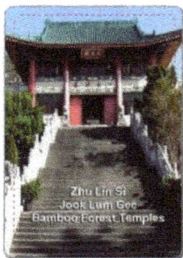
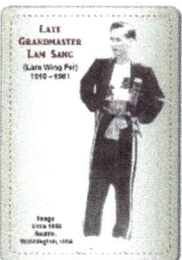
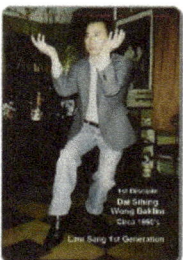
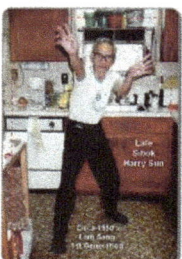
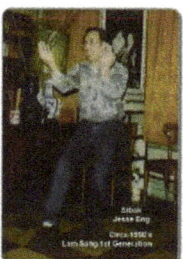

ChinaMantis.com   Instructional DVDs

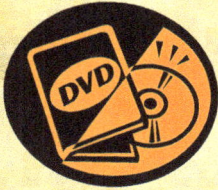

Jook Lum Temple Mantis Step by Step Instruction in 18 Volumes

Year One Training
Volume One: Fundamentals; The Most Important
Volume Two: Phoenix Eye Fist Attacking / Stepping
Volume Three: Centerline Defense
Volume Four: One, Three & Nine Step Attack / Defense
Volume Five: Centerline Sticky Hand Training
Volume Six: Same Hand / Opposite Hand Attacks
Volume Seven: Sai Shu, Sik Shu, Jik (Chun) Shu
Volume Eight: Gow Choy; Hammer Fist-Internal Strength
Volume Nine: Footwork in Southern Praying Mantis
Volume 10 Chi Sao Sticky Hands and Passoffs

Advanced Two Man Forms—Year Two and Three
Available by request. Prerequisite Volumes 1– 10.

Volume 11: Loose Hands One
Volume 12: Som Bo Gin
Volume 13: Second Loose Hands
Volume 14: 108 Subset
Volume 15: Um Hon One
Volume 16: Um Hon Two
Volume 17: Mui Fa Plum Flower
Volume 18: Eighteen Buddha Hands

All 8 two man forms must be trained as one continuous set on both A - B sides.

Summary Year One
http://www.chinamantis.com/first-year-training.htm

Summary Year Three:
http://www.chinamantis.com/summary-of-training.htm

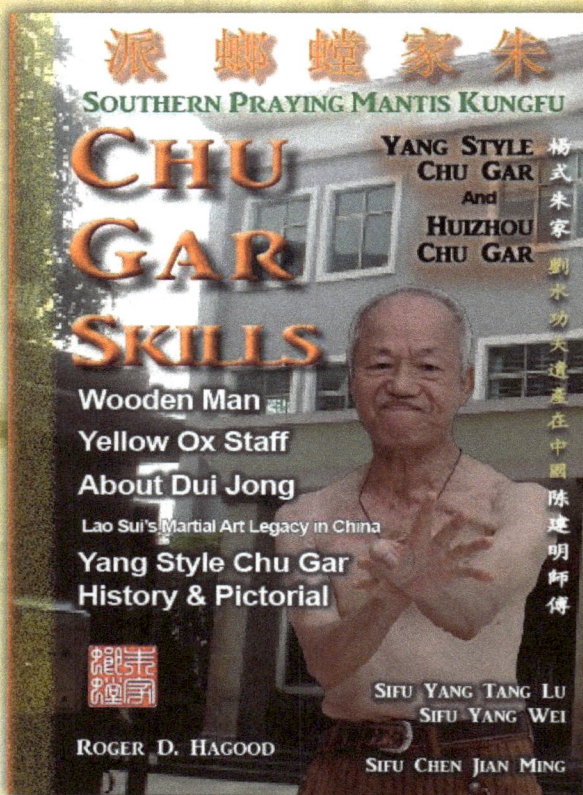

126

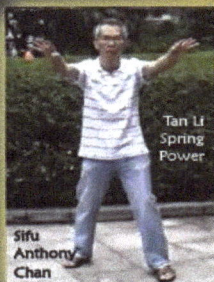

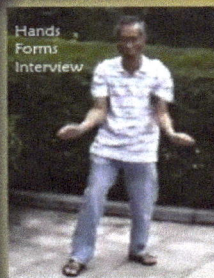

Book Specs
- Hardcover
- 5.5 x 8.5"
- 150 Pages
- 400+ Photographs
- Full Color Interior
- Acid Free Archival Quality

Pictorial of Chu Gar Boxing Skills The complete single man training transmission of 1st Generation late Sifu Chu Kai Ming. 12 Basic Hand Skills, Three Forms. And more.

Visit www.SouthernMantisPress.com

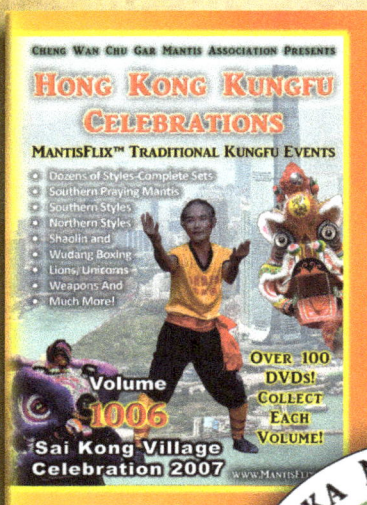

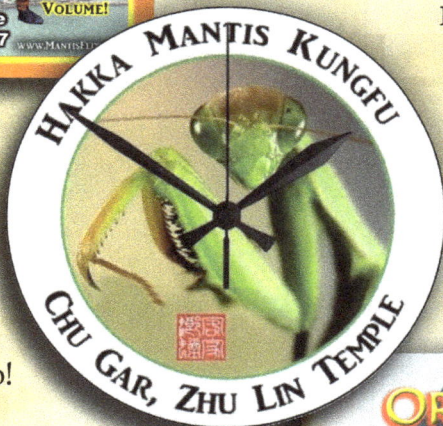

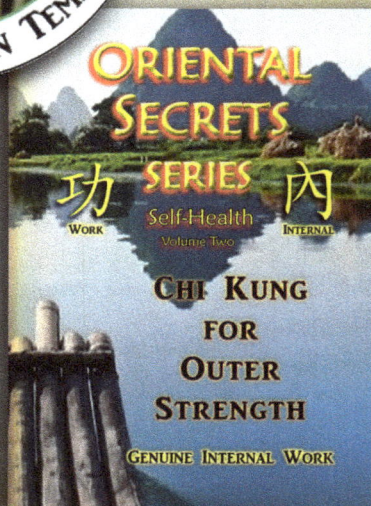

128

RDH Bio

Welcome to visit the Author!

Your email correspondence is welcome and do visit and study Hakka Southern Praying Mantis with me in beautiful sunny south China!   I am an Author, Publisher and Producer of eBooks, books, journals, videos and 7 International martial arts newsstand magazines in 15 countries with 48 years in training and teaching martial arts and some 20+ years living in China and Asia!

Currently residing in beautiful sunny south China for the last 15 years where I teach Southern Praying Mantis.   Join my class in Guangdong today!

RDH
Pingshan Town
Summer 2015

More Bio:
http://www.chinamantis.com/roger-d.-hagood.htm
Email:
rdh@chinamantis.com

Study Hakka Mantis and Unicorn in China

Study in Beautiful South China!

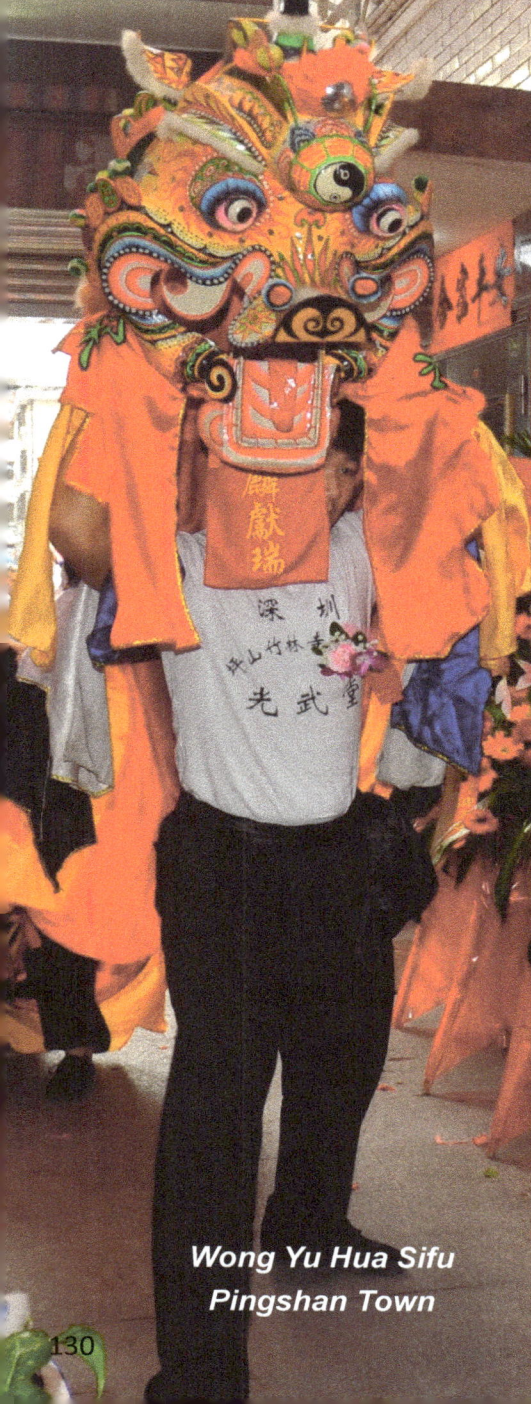

屍舞
獻瑞

深圳
坪山竹林香
光武堂

Train Hakka Unicorn Culture at Guang Wu Tang - The Martial Hall of Wong Yuk Kong! Email your details for consideration today. rdh@chinamantis.com

Wong Yu Hua Sifu
Pingshan Town

www.ingramcontent.com/pod-product-compliance
Lightning Source LLC
Chambersburg PA
CBHW040406110426
42812CB00011B/2471